Urological Cancers in Clinical Practice

Jonathan Waxman (Ed.)

Urological Cancers in Clinical Practice

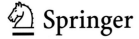 Springer

Jonathan Waxman, BSc, MD, FRCP
Professor of Oncology
Department of Oncology, Division of Surgery, Oncology
Reproductive Biology and Anaesthetics (SORA)
Faculty of Medicine, Imperial College London
The Garry Weston Centre, Hammersmith Hospital, London, UK

Chapters 1–7 and 9–11 reproduced, with updates, from chapters 5, 7, 8, 9, 13, 14, 17, 20, 21, and 24, respectively in: Waxman J. *Urological Cancers*, © 2005 Springer-Verlag London Ltd. Chapter 8 reproduced with modifications, artwork fully reproduced, from chapter 18 in: Waxman J. *Urological Cancers*, © 2005 Springer-Verlag London Ltd.

British Library Cataloguing in Publication Data
A catalogue record for this book is available from the British Library

Library of Congress Control Number: 2006926463

ISBN-10: 1-84628-464-3   e-ISBN 10: 1-84628-507-0   Printed on acid-free paper
ISBN-13: 978-1-84628-464-9   e-ISBN-13: 978-1-84628-507-3

9 8 7 6 5 4 3 2 1

Springer Science+Business Media

springer.com

Preface

Urological cancer is a significant part of modern oncology and urological practice. *Urological Cancers in Clinical Practice* is a companion to *Urological Cancers* which has been recently published by Springer and provides a working guide to the modern management of urological tumours. This is an area where there have been significant changes in treatment in recent times. These changes, which cross the broad spectrum of urological oncology, encompass a huge area of pharmacological development. I hope that *Urological Cancers in Clinical Practice* provides a summary of these developments that enables the practising physician and surgeon to apply the best of the most modern approaches to everyday medical practice.

Jonathan Waxman
London, October 2006

Contents

Contributors

Paul D. Abel, ChM, FRCS
Department of Surgery
Faculty of Medicine
Hammersmith Hospital Campus
Imperial College London
London, UK

Dean F. Bajorin, MD
Genitourinary Medical Oncology Service
Department of Medicine, Solid Tumour Oncology
Memorial Hospital for Cancer and Allied Diseases
Memorial Sloan-Kettering Cancer Center
New York, NY, USA

Simon Chowdhury, MB BS
Department of Medicine
Royal Marsden Hospital
London, UK

Timothy J. Christmas, MD, FRCS(Urol)
Department of Urology
Imperial College School of Medicine
Charing Cross Hospital
London, UK

Gairin J. Dancey, MRCP
Department of Medical Oncology
Charing Cross Hospital
London, UK

Timothy G. Eisen, PhD, FRCP
Renal, Melanoma and Lung Units
Department of Medicine
Royal Marsden Hospital
London, UK

Reena Engineer, DNB
Department of Radiation Oncology
Tata Memorial Hospital
Mumbai, India

Mererid Evans, MB BCh, BSc, PhD, MRCP
Section of Clinical Oncology and Palliative Medicine
University of Wales College of Medicine
Velindre Hospital
Cardiff, UK

Mark R. Feneley, MD, FRCS
Institute of Urology and Nephrology
University College London and UCLH
Foundation Trust
London, UK

Mayer N. Fishman, MD, PhD
Genitourinary Oncology & Experimental Therapeutics
Department of Interdisciplinary Oncology
H. Lee Moffitt Cancer Center and Research Institute
University of South Florida
Tampa, FL, USA

Matthew D. Galsky, MD
Genitourinary Medical Oncology Service
Department of Medicine, Solid Tumour Oncology
Memorial Sloan-Kettering Cancer Center
New York, NY, USA

Thomas R. Geldart, MB BS, BSc, MRCP
Department of Medical Oncology
Southampton General Hospital
Cancer Care Directorate
Southampton, UK

Martin Gore, MB BS, PhD, FRCP
Department of Medical Oncology
Royal Marsden Hospital
London, UK

Roger S. Kirby, MA, MD, FRCS
The Prostate Centre
London, UK

Malcolm D. Mason, MD, FRCP, FRCR
Section of Clinical Oncology and Palliative Medicine
University of Wales College of Medicine
Velindre Hospital
Cardiff, UK

Graham M. Mead, DM, FRCP, FRCR
Department of Medical Oncology
Southampton General Hospital
Cancer Care Directorate
Southampton, UK

Malcolm J. Moore, MD
Department of Medical Oncology and Hematology
Princess Margaret Hospital
University Health Network
Toronto, ON, Canada

Jeremy L. Ockrim, MD, BSc, FRCS
Department of Urology
Institute of Urology
University College London
London, UK

Rajiv Sarin, MD, FRCR
Advanced Centre for Treatment, Research & Education in
    Cancer (ACTREC)
Tata Memorial Centre
Mumbai, India

Gillian L. Smith, MD, FRCS
Department of Urology
The Royal Free Hospital
London, UK

Srikala S. Sridhar, MD, MSc
Department of Medicine
McMaster University
Juravinski Cancer Centre
Hamilton, ON, Canada

Hemant B. Tongaonkar, MS
Genitourinary and Gynaecological Services
Tata Memorial Hospital
Mumbai, India

Jonathan Waxman, BSc, MD, FRCP
Department of Oncology
Division of Surgery, Oncology, Reproductive Biology and
    Anaesthetics (SORA)
Faculty of Medicine
Imperial College London
Hammersmith Hospital
London, UK

1

Radical Radiotherapy for Prostate Cancer

Mererid Evans and Malcolm D. Mason

Key Points

1. There have been no randomised trials comparing brachytherapy or IMRT with conventional radiotherapy.
2. ADJUVANT radiotherapy has recently been shown to improve progression-free survival after radical surgery in patients with tumour at excision margins or infiltrating seminal vesicles.
3. Hormone therapy improves outcomes (progression free survival and survival) after radical radiotherapy for locally advanced disease.

Introduction

The incidence of prostate cancer is rising worldwide due to the ageing of the population and the increasing availability of prostate-specific antigen (PSA) screening. Prostate-specific antigen testing has led specifically to an increase in the proportion of patients diagnosed with early-stage (localized) prostate cancer. Radical radiotherapy is one of the curative treatment options for localized prostate cancer and it also has a role to play in locally advanced and even metastatic disease. This chapter reviews the relative merits of radiotherapy in comparison to the other management options for early prostate cancer and summarizes the staggering technological advances that have occurred in prostate radiotherapy over the last decade.

Treatment of Early (Localized) Prostate Cancer

The Role of Radical Radiotherapy

The optimum management of patients with localized prostate cancer remains controversial. Three major treatment options are available: radical prostatectomy, radical radiotherapy (external beam radiotherapy [EBRT] or brachytherapy), and active surveillance (also known as active monitoring and watchful waiting). Each treatment involves its own risk. Radical treatments can cause harmful side effects including incontinence, erectile dysfunction, and even death, whereas watchful waiting causes anxiety relating to the presence of cancer and carries a risk of disease progression. However, outcomes in terms of overall survival appear similar with each of the three modalities.

There is relatively little randomized evidence concerning the effectiveness of the different management options for early prostate cancer. In a Scandinavian study [1], men with early prostate cancer (stages T1b-c or T2) were randomly assigned to radical prostatectomy or watchful waiting. After a median follow-up of 6.2 years, there was a significant reduction in disease-specific mortality in the radical prostatectomy group compared with the watchful waiting group (4.6% vs. 8.9%, $P = .02$), but there was no significant difference in overall survival between the two groups. A randomized trial comparing surgery with radiotherapy published in 1982 showed better survival outcomes in the surgery group [2]. However, this was a small (97 patients), single-center trial conducted in the pre-PSA era, and it is unlikely to be relevant to contemporary practice. Unfortunately, a United Kingdom Medical Research Council (MRC) trial (PR06) randomizing patients to radical prostatectomy, radical radiotherapy, and watchful waiting was closed in 1997 because of poor recruitment, which was attributed to an unwillingness among participants and clinicians to accept randomization.

A number of nonrandomized, retrospective studies have compared the outcomes of the different treatment modalities for early prostate cancer. A study from Boston compared outcomes in 2254 men treated with radical prostatectomy and 381 men treated with conventional dose (66 Gy) radiotherapy [3]. There was a possible advantage for surgery in low-risk patients, but no difference between treatment modalities in intermediate or high-risk cases. Another study from the Cleveland Clinic compared outcomes in 1054 men who underwent radical prostatectomy and 628 treated with radiotherapy [4]. When stratified by prognostic risk groups, there was no difference in biochemical control between patients undergoing prostatectomy and patients having radiotherapy to dose levels ≥72 Gy; however, the outcome of patients who received lower-dose radiotherapy was less favorable. There are many problems with retrospective comparisons like these, including differences in case selection and length of follow-up, and the inherent disadvantages of analyzing past rather than contemporary practice.

At least two large randomized trials are currently in progress, although their results are not yet available. The United States Prostate Cancer Intervention Versus Observation Trial (PIVOT) is comparing radical prostatectomy and watchful waiting for localized prostate cancer [5]; it opened in 1994 and has now closed to recruitment. The U.K. Protect study (*Pro*state *Te*sting for *C*ancer and *T*reatment) combines the identification of men with prostate cancer detected by PSA screening with a randomized trial comparing radical prostatectomy, radical EBRT, and watchful waiting. The issue of randomization to the various treatment options was successfully addressed in a feasibility study, which has aided recruitment into this study, and has shown that with careful management, it is possible to randomize prostate cancer patients into trials such as this.

While the results of these studies are awaited, clinical decision making in early prostate cancer should be tailored to the individual patient and take account of tumor prognosis (Gleason grade, stage, and PSA), background health, life expectancy, and patient preference. It is common to offer curative treatment to men who have a life expectancy of 10 years or more and to consider treatment for men with a life expectancy of 5 years or more if the tumor is poorly differentiated. Treatment-related morbidity and quality-of-life issues are important considerations and patients should be counseled appropriately. Prostatectomy patients are significantly more likely than radiotherapy patients to experience urinary incontinence (39% to 49% vs. 6% to 7%) and erectile dysfunction (80% to 91% vs. 41% to 55%), whereas radiotherapy patients are more likely to experience bowel urgency (30% to 35% vs. 6% to 7%) [6].

Standard External Beam Radiotherapy (EBRT)

Radical EBRT is an alternative to radical prostatectomy for patients with early, organ-confined prostate cancer (T1-2, N0, M0) and can also be used for patients with nonmetastatic locally advanced disease (T3-T4) where surgery is inappropriate.

Pretreatment Assessment

The primary tumor is assessed by digital rectal examination, cystoscopy, and transrectal ultrasound (TRUS). Staging of systemic disease usually comprises bone scanning and pelvic lymph node imaging (with computed tomography [CT] or magnetic resonance imaging [MRI]), although these investigations are sometimes omitted in patients with particularly "good risk" features. Magnetic resonance imaging scanning is particularly useful in assessing capsular invasion, seminal vesicle involvement, and periapical extension, and can aid treatment planning.

Treatment Planning

Computed tomography planning is now standard practice in most U.K. centers. Prior to the advent of CT planning, the size and position of the prostate was indirectly visualized using a cystourethrogram, putting barium in the rectum and taking orthogonal films, upon which the target volume could be drawn. The target volume is usually defined as the prostate plus all/base of the seminal vesicles, or any grossly visible tumor, with a margin of 1 to 1.5 cm to allow for microscopic spread and for variations in treatment setup (Fig. 1.1). A smaller margin is often allowed at the rectal–prostate interface if there is too much rectum in the high-dose volume. In the absence of macroscopic disease in the seminal vesicles, there is some debate as to whether they should be included in the treatment volume or not. Simple formulas for predicting the probability of microscopic seminal vesicle involvement based on the T stage, Gleason score, and pretreatment PSA level can be helpful.

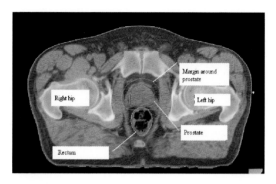

Fig. 1.1. Computed tomography (CT) scan through the center of the target volume showing the rectum, femoral heads, prostate (or clinical target volume, CTV), and a margin around the prostate to be treated to high dose (the planning target volume, PTV).

Inconsistencies in treatment volume definition occur among clinicians [7], especially in outlining the prostatic apex, superior aspect of the prostate projecting into the bladder, seminal vesicles, the base of the seminal vesicles, and superior rectum. These should be considered when designing and comparing trials of radiotherapy.

Technique

Patients are treated in the supine position with a full bladder (this helps push bowel out of the high-dose area), once daily, 5 days a week. Skin tattoos are placed anteriorly over the pubic symphysis and laterally over the iliac crests to aid treatment setup. Three-field techniques using an anterior and two posterior oblique fields are commonly used, although four- and even six-field techniques are used in some centers (Fig. 1.2).

Dose and Fractionation

The optimum dose and fractionation schedule for EBRT is unclear. Until recently, standard treatment schedules in many centers delivered daily fractions of 1.8 to 2 Gy per day, to a total dose upwards of 64 Gy.

There is evidence that the α/β ratio for prostate cancer may be as low as 1.5, comparable to late-responding normal tissues,

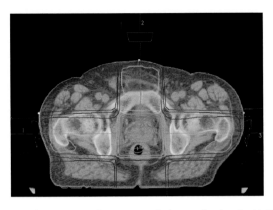

Fig. 1.2. Three-field technique for prostate radiotherapy showing the 10, 20, 50, 70, 90, 95, 100, and 102 isodoses. The CTV, PTV, and rectum are outlined.

probably because of the slow turnover rate of prostate tumors [8]. This suggests that prostate cancers may be particularly sensitive to hypofractionation and that using larger fraction sizes could result in greater cell kill. In addition to the possible radiobiological gains, other benefits to hypofractionation include shorter overall treatment times and a smaller number of hospital visits, which increases patient convenience and reduces resource utilization.

The outcome of 705 men with T1-4 prostate cancer treated in Manchester with conformal, hypofractionated radiotherapy (50 Gy in 16 daily fractions) has been analyzed [9]. The 5-year biochemical-free survival rates for good, intermediate, and poor prognostic groups were 82%, 56%, and 39%, respectively, which are comparable to published results using conventional fractionation, and normal tissue toxicity rates were not increased. The results of the first randomized study of hypofractionated radiotherapy for localized prostate cancer were presented at the 45th annual meeting of the American Society for Therapeutic Radiology and Oncology (ASTRO) [10]; 936 patients with T1/T2 prostate cancer were randomized at 16 Canadian centers to receive either 66 Gy in 33 fractions over $6\frac{1}{2}$ weeks or 52.5 Gy in 20 fractions over 4 weeks. After a median follow-up of 59 months, the treatment failure rate appeared to be slightly higher in the hypofractionated arm than in the conventional arm, but there was no significant difference between the two groups in biopsy positivity 2 years after radiotherapy or in overall survival (with a trend for both in favor of the hypofractionated arm). Also, although acute toxicity was higher in the hypofractionated group, late toxicity was similar in both groups.

The development of conformal radiotherapy has led to a surge of interest in dose escalation (above 70 Gy), which is discussed later in the chapter.

Toxicity

The side effects of EBRT can be divided into acute and late reactions. Acute reactions start about halfway through a course of treatment and principally involve the bladder (cystitis) and bowel (proctitis, occasional enteritis). These effects normally settle with conservative management within 4 to 6 weeks of the end of treatment. Rarely, severe acute side effects may necessitate a break in treatment, but it is unusual for acute effects to be dose limiting in practice. It is rare for patients to experience significant skin toxicity with EBRT, though a reaction is not infrequently seen superior to the natal cleft due to the exit dose from the anterior beam in a three-field arrangement.

Late side effects are generally more "dose- limiting" than acute effects because they can have a significant impact on quality of life and are often permanent. They may appear between 6 months and 2 years after radiotherapy, although sometimes acute effects do not settle and can continue as late effects. Late urogenital toxicity manifests as chronic cystitis, urinary incontinence (2% to 11%) and erectile dysfunction (10% to 40%). Late damage to the rectum results in late radiation proctitis, rectal ulceration, or stricture; severe damage occasionally necessitates a defunctioning colostomy (risk <1%).

Efficacy

The outcome of patients treated with modern, high-dose radiotherapy is comparable to surgery, at least over a 5-year period. Five-year actuarial biochemical relapse-free survival rates of 90% have been reported for favorable risk patients treated with >75 Gy [11]. Pretreatment PSA level, Gleason score, tumor stage, radiation dose (<70 Gy or ≥70 Gy), and treatment year are all significant prognostic factors. The posttreatment PSA nadir has been found to be highly predictive of outcome; in one study, 75% of patients with a PSA nadir of <0.5 ng/mL had PSA disease-free survival (DFS) at 8 years compared to only 12% of patients with a PSA nadir >4 ng/mL [12].

Three-Dimensional Conformal Radiotherapy (3D-CRT)

Conventional radiotherapy is delivered using rectangular-shaped treatment fields, which inevitably encompass large volumes of normal tissues as well as the required target volume. The major focus over the last decade has been the development of conformal radiotherapy techniques, which allow delivery of irregularly shaped fields that conform more closely to the tumor target while reducing the radiation to the dose-limiting normal tissues. Shaping of fields can be achieved in one of two ways: by putting a custom-made lead shield in front of the beam, or by making the beam itself irregular in shape by using multileaf collimators (MLCs) (Fig. 1.3).

Does Conformal Radiotherapy Reduce Toxicity?

A randomized study comparing conventional and conformal radiotherapy at a standard dose of 64 Gy [13] showed a significant reduction in late (>3 months after treatment) radiation-induced proctitis and bleeding in the conformal group compared with the conventional group (5% vs. 15%, Radiation Therapy Oncology Group [RTOG] grade 2 or higher, $p = .01$). There were no differences between groups in bladder function after treatment. After a median follow-up of 3.6 years, there was no significant difference between groups in local tumor control: conformal 78% (95% confidence interval [CI] 66–86); conventional 83% (95% CI 69–90). These results have provided the basis for dose-escalation studies in an attempt to improve local tumor control with acceptable toxicity.

Fig. 1.3. (a) Beam's-eye view of right lateral treatment field for conformal prostate radiotherapy. Field shaping has been achieved by the use of multileaf collimators (MLCs) (shown in yellow). The collimator angle has been optimized to conform to the posterior edge of the PTV (shown in red) to protect the rectum. (b) The multileaf collimator.

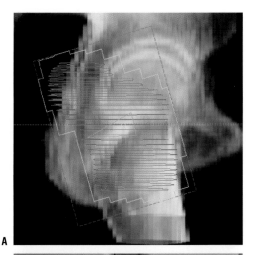

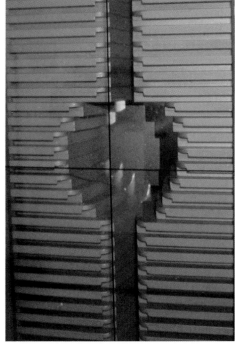

Dose Escalation

In a randomized dose-escalation trial conducted at the M.D. Anderson Cancer Center, 305 men with localized (T1 to T3) prostate cancer were randomized to receive either conventional-dose (70 Gy) or high-dose (78 Gy) conformal radiotherapy to the prostate and seminal vesicles [14]. With a median follow-up of 60 months, the biochemical control rates at 6 years were significantly higher in the 78-Gy arm compared to the 70-Gy arm (70% vs. 64%, $p = .03$). Subgroup analysis suggested that the benefit of dose escalation was limited to patients with a pretreatment PSA of $\geqslant 10$ ng/mL (biochemical control rate, 62% vs. 43%, $p = .01$) but that there was no significant dose response in patients who had a pretreatment PSA of ≤ 10 ng/mL. The trial did not show a significant effect of dose escalation on overall survival, although there was a trend toward a higher freedom from distant metastasis rate at 6 years in patients with PSA levels >10 ng/mL who were treated with 78 Gy (98% vs. 88%, $p = .056$). Rectal side effects were significantly greater in the 78-Gy group (grade 2 rectal toxicity rates at 6 years, 26% vs. 12%, $p = .001$), whereas the rate of bladder complications was similar in both arms. The risk of rectal toxicity correlated highly with the proportion of the rectum treated to >70 Gy, and it was suggested by the authors that the rectal volume receiving ≥ 70 Gy should be limited to <25% in future dose escalation trials. The ongoing RTOG 94-06 trial is attempting to establish the maximum tolerated dose that can be delivered to the prostate using 3D-CRT. Interim results for patients treated to 79.2 Gy using 1.8-Gy fractions have demonstrated low levels of toxicity [15], and the study has continued using 2-Gy fractions to dose levels of 74 and 78 Gy.

The M.D. Anderson data are supported by data from a number of retrospective and prospective PSA-era trials that have provided evidence for a dose response in prostate cancer. However, more studies are required to define the groups of patients who may benefit from dose escalation and to assess whether there is any benefit in terms of survival. It is possible that conventional doses are sufficient in low-risk patients and that dose escalation may just increase toxicity with no benefit in terms of disease control in these patients. The results of several randomized trials of dose escalation in the UK, the Netherlands, France, and North America are awaited. The UK MRC RT01 trial, which randomized men to standard-dose (64 Gy) or high-dose (74 Gy) con-

formal radiotherapy in addition to neoadjuvant androgen suppression, closed to accrual in 2001 with around 800 patients
randomized.

Intensity-Modulated Radiotherapy

Intensity-modulated radiotherapy (IMRT) is an advanced
form of 3D-CRT that allows tighter conformation to the
target volume and sparing of normal tissues in the vicinity of and
even within the target volume to an extent that was not previously
possible. In general, IMRT uses inverse treatment planning
systems that work backward from a desired dose distribution
to generate treatment fields with varying intensities across the
cross section of the beam. Treatment delivery utilizes MLCs
where each set of opposing leaves travel across the beam under
computer control during radiation delivery according to a prescribed scheme, to produce the required intensity pattern across
the beam.

Early toxicity and biochemical outcomes have been reported
for 772 patients with localized prostate cancer treated with high-
dose IMRT (81 to 86.4 Gy, 1.8 Gy/fraction) at the Memorial Sloan-
Kettering Cancer Center [16]. Intensity-modulated radiotherapy
was associated with decreased rectal toxicity, and the actuarial
rate of grade ≥2 proctitis at 3 years was only 4% compared to the
rate of 14% previously reported at the same center for patients
receiving 81 Gy with 3D-CRT [11]. The 3-year actuarial PSA
relapse-free survival rates were comparable to published results
using 3D-CRT; however, median follow-up was only 24 months
and longer follow-up is required to substantiate these results.
Preliminary results using hypofractionated IMRT (70 Gy at
2.5 Gy/fraction) show similar rates of late toxicity and biochemical outcome to high-dose 3D-CRT [17], although again, longer
follow-up is required.

Although prophylactic pelvic lymph node radiotherapy is not
routine practice in the U.K., there is evidence from the RTOG
9413 study that it may be beneficial in carefully selected patients
[18]. The potential of IMRT to irradiate pelvic lymph nodes while
sparing critical pelvic organs has been investigated [19]. Conventional radiotherapy plans were compared to 3D-CRT and
IMRT plans for 10 patients. The mean percentage volume of
small bowel receiving >45 Gy for the conventional radiotherapy,
3D-CRT, and IMRT plans were 21%, 18%, and 5%, respectively,

($p < .001$). The rectal and bladder volumes irradiated with doses ≥ 45 Gy were also reduced by IMRT. The reduction in critical pelvic organ irradiation seen with IMRT may reduce side effects and allow modest dose escalation. A phase I dose-escalation trial has been initiated to assess the tolerance of radiotherapy to the pelvic lymph nodes of 50 to 60 Gy using IMRT.

Concerns have been raised that reducing treatment volumes to such an extent carries a risk of incurring a geographical miss of the target, which would inevitably result in reduced tumour control. However, results so far suggest that PSA outcomes after IMRT are comparable to conventional 3D-CRT, although mature data are not yet available. Other potential drawbacks to IMRT include the added workload on physicians, physicists, and radiotherapists, the risk of errors due to the complexity of planning and delivery, and the complexity of quality assurance. An additional concern is that IMRT may lead to an increase in the incidence of second malignancies. There are two reasons for this: (1) IMRT involves the use of more fields than conventional radiotherapy and, as a consequence, a larger volume of normal tissues is exposed to low radiation doses; (2) IMRT usually requires more time to deliver a specified dose than conventional radiotherapy (hence more monitor units needed) thus increasing the total body exposure, due to leakage radiation. Careful long-term follow-up of patients treated with IMRT is necessary to address this issue.

Prostate Brachytherapy

Prostate brachytherapy involves placement of radioactive sources directly into the parenchyma of the prostate. It is a highly conformal form of therapy, permitting dose escalation to the target volume far exceeding that of other radiation modalities. The surrounding normal tissues are spared because of the rapid dose falloff with distance from the source (inverse square law). The evolution of TRUS imaging, a closed transperineal approach, and the increasing sophistication of computerized planning have resulted in a worldwide resurgence of interest in this treatment technique. Its appeal lies in its speed and convenience (it can be done as an outpatient procedure) and the low long-term risk of proctitis; impotence is also less likely than after radical prostatectomy. Brachytherapy to the prostate can be delivered either with permanent seed implants or with removable implants, which are often delivered at a high dose rate with iridium wire.

Permanent Implants

Permanent implants may be used alone as monotherapy for localized prostate cancer or, less commonly, as a boost in combination with EBRT. Patient selection is extremely important for two reasons: (1) to identify patients who are likely to have a good outcome in terms of biochemical disease free survival, and (2) to identify patients who will have a good functional outcome. Patients who are likely to have a good outcome from brachytherapy alone have an initial PSA level <10 ng/mL, Gleason score ≤6, and low-volume disease with a low risk of extracapsular spread (stage T1/T2). If the prostate is large (>50 cm^3), the pubic rami may shield part of the gland that cannot be adequately implanted; these patients also need a large number of seeds and are at increased risk of morbidity. If otherwise suitable, neoadju- vant hormone treatment with a luteinizing hormone–releasing hormone (LHRH) analogue for 3 months can lead to a reduction in prostate volume of >30%. Brachytherapy should be avoided in men with a history of transurethral resection of the prostate (TURP) because it increases the risk of long-term urinary incontinence following brachytherapy from 1% to ~12.5%. An alternative procedure may also be preferable in patients with significant pretreatment lower urinary tract obstructive symptoms who are more likely to develop urinary retention after brachytherapy.

Two isotopes are used as the radioactive seed source, iodine (^{125}I) and palladium (^{103}Pd), although only ^{125}I is readily obtainable in the U.K. Both isotopes have low energy but different half-lives (59.4 days for ^{125}I, 16.97 days for ^{103}Pd) and initial dose rate. ^{103}Pd has the higher dose rate and is biologically more active; therefore, equivalent prescribed doses are lower. For patients treated by brachytherapy alone, typical doses are 145 Gy with ^{125}I and 100 Gy with ^{103}Pd, which is the minimum peripheral dose to the margin of the target volume. If brachytherapy is used in conjunction with EBRT, typically prescribed doses are 45 Gy in 25 fractions given by EBRT followed by 110 Gy via an ^{125}I-brachytherapy implant [20].

A two-stage technique is most commonly used for permanent implantation in the U.K. The initial stage requires a preplanning TRUS examination performed with the patient in the lithotomy position, done either as an outpatient or day-hospital procedure under general anesthesia. The TRUS images are digitized to produce a 3D model of the prostate on the planning computer, which can be used to determine the num- ber and position of seeds required. The implant is performed a few weeks later in an identical lithotomy position. Thin needles are inserted percuta- neously into the prostate through a perineal template to a precal- culated depth guided by an ultrasound probe in the rectum. The needles may either be preloaded with the appropriate number of seeds or the seeds can be inserted individually. Between 20 and 30 needles containing 60 to 120 seeds are implanted depending on the volume and seed activity. The needles are then removed, leaving the seeds permanently in place. A CT scan is performed after implantation to identify the seeds and prostatic outline, and this information is used to calculate the actual dose delivered to the prostate.

Almost all patients develop urethritis of variable intensity which may last for ~3 months. Symptoms may be helped by alpha-blockers and nonsteroidal antiinflammatory drugs. A minority of patients (15%) develop acute retention either immediately or in the few days following implantation. This is usually due to postimplant edema and requires catheterization. In most patients, micturition resumes within 2 weeks as edema resolves, although recovery may occasionally take longer. Long-term effects include persistent cystitis and prostatitis (3%), proctitis (2%), and impotence (25%). The risk of urinary incontinence is small (~1%) unless patients have had a previous TURP.

There have been no randomized trials comparing brachyther-apy with other interventions for early prostate cancer (though a trial randomizing patients to brachytherapy or radical prostate-ctomy is now open, under the auspices of the American College of Surgeons). Most results come from single centers reporting ret-rospective series [e.g., 21]. These results are extremely promising, but what is difficult to gauge is the extent to which such results reflect the benefit of brachytherapy per se, and to what extent they reflect patient selection factors. Some workers advocate EBRT in conjunction with brachytherapy for patients with intermediate and high risk factors, but it is not yet proven whether this improves outcome.

High Dose Rate Brachytherapy

Remote afterloading systems can also be used with TRUS and template guidance to deliver temporary, high dose rate (HDR) brachytherapy to the prostate. The isotope used is iridium (^{192}Ir), which has higher emission energies than ^{125}I and ^{103}Pd. The greater range may be more suitable for the treatment of patients with bulkier tumors and the possibility of extracapsular extension. Treatment is hypofractionated (with the potential benefits of hypofractionation previously discussed) and treatment times are a few minutes only. Most trials investigating the usefulness of HDR to date have given it as a boost (8 to 10 Gy × 2) prior to, during, or after EBRT (45 to 50 Gy) with good results even in patients with unfavorable prostate cancer [22]. More recently, a number of HDR monotherapy trials [e.g., 23] have shown that the treatment is feasible and well tolerated, but longer follow-up is required for outcome.

Combined Radiotherapy and Hormone Therapy

The use of combined modality treatment, with hormone therapy and radiotherapy, for the treatment of prostate cancer may be beneficial for two reasons. First, by combining two effective modalities, there is hope that the anticancer effects will be additive. Second, the use of hormone therapy to shrink a large prostate before irradiation may improve efficacy by reducing the tumor burden and also may reduce rectal toxicity by reducing the volume irradiated to high dose [24]. The LHRH agonists (e.g., goserelin) are usually used, but antiandrogens (e.g., bicalutamide) may be useful in men who wish to retain their potency, although they result in less prostate shrinkage [25].

The combination of hormone therapy and radiotherapy has been tested in a number of clinical trials with some variation in the way in which hormone therapy was administered (Table 1.1). Based on these findings, there do appear to be several subsets of prostate cancer patients who benefit from hormone therapy plus radiotherapy over radiotherapy alone:

1. Patients with bulky tumors without evidence of distant metastases and Gleason score ≤6 benefit from short-course neoadjuvant hormone therapy for 4 months (2 months before and 2 months during radiotherapy). It is not known if an LHRH

agonist alone would produce the same benefit as the combination of LHRH agonist and antiandrogen used in RTOG 86-10.

2. Patients with any T stage and no evidence of distant metastases with Gleason score 8 to 10 tumors benefit from long-term hormone therapy (2 to 3 years). Periods of 2 to 3 years have been chosen empirically in most trials, but it is possible that a shorter course may be equally effective; the European Organization for Research and Treatment of Cancer (EORTC) trial 22961 is investigating this possibility.

3. At least some patients with T3 tumors and lower Gleason grade also appear to benefit from long-term hormone therapy, based on a meta-analysis of the RTOG protocols [33], and the EORTC study [29].

The potential benefits of androgen deprivation have to be balanced against toxicity. Most patients experience hot flushes, fatigue, and impotence of varying degrees, which can impact significantly on quality of life. Other toxicities include loss of libido, weight gain, muscle wasting, and changes in texture of hair and skin. Longer-term concerns include the development of osteoporosis and the possibility that low testosterone levels may predispose to cardiovascular disease. There is no evidence yet that long-term hormone therapy increases non–prostate cancer mortality, but this is being investigated; in the meantime, it is sensible to restrict the use of long-term hormone therapy to patient groups in which it has been shown to have an overall survival benefit.

None of the trials in Table 1.1 included a hormone therapy alone arm. Because of this, it is not possible to say with certainty whether the benefits that appear in the patients treated with combined modality therapy are due to the combination of radiotherapy and androgen ablation or the androgen ablation *per se*. The MRC PR02 study [34] did include a hormones-alone arm and randomized 277 patients with T2 to T4 prostate cancer and no bone metastases to orchidectomy alone, radiotherapy alone, or a combination of the two. The study was too small to detect a statistically significant difference in overall survival between the groups, but there was a delay in time to metastasis in patients treated with hormone therapy (with or without radiotherapy). A randomized Medical Research Council study (MRC Prof) is investigating whether radiotherapy contributes anything to long-term hormone therapy in patients with nonmetastatic locally advanced or poor prognosis organ-confined prostate cancer.

Table 1.1. Randomized trials of hormone therapy plus radiotherapy

Study	Patient numbers	Patient characteristics	Timing	Outcome
RTOG 85–31 [26,27]	977	T3 or LN positive	Adjuvant goserelin, last week of RT until progression	↑ LC, ↓ DM but OS NS except in Gleason 8 to 10
EORTC [28,29]	415	T1–2 grade 3 or T3–4, any grade (LN negative)	Adjuvant goserelin, first week of RT for 3 years	↑ DFS and OS at 5 years
RTOG 86–10 [30]	471	Bulky T2–4 (+/– LN positive)	Neoadjuvant CAS, 2 months before and 2 months during RT	Overall, ↑ LC, ↓ DM but not in Gleason 7 to 10; OS NS except in Gleason 2 to 6
RTOG 92–02 [31]	1554	T2C–T4, PSA <150 ng/mL	Neoadjuvant CAS for 2 months before +2 months during RT for all patients, then adjuvant goserelin for 2 years or no further treatment	↑ LC, ↑ DFS, ↓ DM but OS NS except in Gleason 8 to 10
RTOG 94–13 [18,32]	1323	T1–4 with risk LN positive >15% or T2C–T4 Gleason ≥6 even if risk LN positive <15%	2 × 2 design: whole pelvic vs. prostate RT; neoadjuvant CAS for 2 months before +2 months during RT; CAS for 4 months after RT.	↑ PFS for whole pelvic + neoadjuvant hormones but OS NS during RT or adjuvant

CAS, combined androgen suppression (goserelin + flutamide); DFS, disease-free survival; DM, distant metastases; EORTC, European Organization for Research and Treatment of Cancer; LC, local control; LN, lymph node; NS, nonsignificant; OS, overall survival; PFS, progression free survival; RT, radiotherapy; RTOG, Radiation Therapy Oncology Group.

Adjuvant or Salvage Radiotherapy After Surgery

Following radical prostatectomy, patients with positive resection margins, extraprostatic extension (pT3 disease), or seminal vesicle invasion are at increased risk of disease recurrence. There is increasing interest in the role of postoperative radiotherapy in these patients. Radiotherapy (RT) can be administered immediately following prostatectomy (adjuvant RT) or may be postponed until the PSA has risen to a level that is indicative of residual or recurrent prostate cancer (salvage RT). There are no published randomized clinical trials of postprostatectomy radiotherapy, and it is not known whether the results of immediate adjuvant radiotherapy and early salvage radiotherapy are equivalent. Most retrospective studies, however, show that both are generally well tolerated.

Adjuvant radiotherapy is given postoperatively to eradicate possible microscopic residual disease in the periprostatic tissues or adjacent pelvic lymph nodes. It may be considered in men with positive resection margins, extraprostatic extension, or an elevated PSA after surgery. Retrospective studies show that it reduces the local and biochemical recurrence rates in high-risk patients after radical prostatectomy, but there is no evidence yet that it improves survival [35]. Seminal vesicle invasion predicts biochemical failure (rise in PSA) after adjuvant radiotherapy, presumably because it is associated with a high risk of distant metastases. The results of two completed, but yet to be reported, randomized trials of postoperative radiotherapy are awaited in the near future. The Southwest Oncology Group (SWOG) 8794 trial and EORTC 22911 trial have randomized a combined total of over 1300 patients with unfavorable prostate cancer to receive either adjuvant radiotherapy or observation (with salvage radiation on recurrence) following radical prostatectomy.

Salvage radiotherapy is given for patients with biochemical or clinical evidence of recurrent disease following prostatectomy. This approach spares ~40% of patients with high-risk features postprostatectomy who may never have a recurrence. Only patients with disease recurrence confined to the prostatic bed are likely to benefit, and it is therefore important to determine whether a rising PSA represents local recurrence or whether it is an indicator of metastatic disease. Even with local-only recurrence, salvage radiation may not be necessary if life expectancy is short and the risk of symptomatic prostate cancer is low. This is supported by a study of patients with biochemical failure following prostatectomy from Johns Hopkins University, in which the median time from biochemical failure to detection of metastases was 8 years, and the median time from detection of metastases to death was 5 years [36].

Response rates after salvage radiotherapy vary between 10% and 76%, with different patient selection criteria being the most likely explanation for the enormous difference between studies. Factors that predict a favorable outcome after salvage radiotherapy include low preradiation PSA level, low Gleason grade, absence of seminal vesicle involvement, and biochemical failure to be consistent >1 year after prostatectomy [37]. Presalvage PSA appears to be the most consistently reported prognostic variable, and salvage rates are low for patients with pre-RT PSA >2 ng/mL. The increasing sensitivity of PSA testing means that salvage radiotherapy can now be started at much lower PSA levels (0.01 to 0.1 ng/mL) with the expectation that this will yield better results. Consequently, trials using salvage radiotherapy for men with higher PSA levels (including SWOG 8794 and EORTC 22911) may therefore underestimate the efficacy of early salvage radiotherapy compared to adjuvant radiotherapy, and this needs to be considered in their interpretation.

The role of hormone therapy in combination with postoperative radiotherapy is currently unknown. Two RTOG studies currently in progress are addressing this issue: RTOG P-0011 is comparing adjuvant radiotherapy alone versus adjuvant combined modality therapy in high-risk postprostatectomy patients, whereas RTOG 9601 is comparing salvage radiotherapy alone versus combined modality therapy in patients with a rising PSA (>0.2 ng/mL and <4 ng/mL) after radical prostatectomy.

Conclusion

Current evidence suggests that radiotherapy is as effective as other curative modalities for prostate cancer. As well as the need for more mature data from high-dose, conformal studies, the ongoing randomized trials will better define its role. The optimum duration of hormone therapy is still unclear, and the patient population that most benefits from combined hormone therapy plus radiotherapy needs to be better defined. The next 5 to 10 years will yield some important data in clarifying these and other issues.

Controversies and Outstanding Issues

1. Does radical radiotherapy prevent progression to metastatic disease?
2. Does increasing the radiotherapy treatment dose increase local control rates?

References

1. Holmberg L, Bill-Axelson A, Helgesen F, et al. A randomised trial comparing radical prostatectomy with watchful waiting in early prostate cancer. N Engl J Med 2002;347:781–789.
2. Paulson DF, Lin GH, Hinshaw W, et al. Radical surgery versus radiotherapy for adenocarcinoma of the prostate. J Urol 1982;128:502–504.
3. D'Amico AV, Whittington R, Malcowicz SB, et al. Biochemical outcome after radical prostatectomy or external beam radiation therapy for patients with clinically localised prostate carcinoma in the prostate specific antigen era. Cancer 2002;95:281–286.
4. Kupelian PA, Elshaikh M, Reddy CA, et al. Comparison of the efficacy of local therapies for localised prostate cancer in the prostate-specific antigen era: a large single-institution experience with radical prostatectomy and external-beam radiotherapy. J Clin Oncol 2002; 20:3376–3385.
5. Wilt TJ, Brawer MK. The prostate cancer intervention versus observation trial; a randomised trial comparing radical prostatectomy versus expectant management for the treatment of clinically localised prostate cancer. J Urol 1994;152:1910–1914.
6. Madalinska JB, Essink-Bot M-L, de Koning HJ, et al. Health-related quality-of-life effects of radical prostatectomy and primary radiotherapy for screen-detected or clinically diagnosed localised prostate cancer. J Clin Oncol 2001;19: 1619–1628.
7. Seddon B, Bidmead M, Wilson J, et al. Target volume definition in conformal radiotherapy for prostate cancer: quality assurance in the MRC RT-01 trial. Radiother Oncol 2000;56:73–83.
8. Brenner DJ, Hall EJ. Fractionation and protraction for radiotherapy of prostate carcinoma. Int J Radiat Oncol Biol Phys 1999;43:1095–1101.
9. Livsey JE, Cowan RA, Wylie JP, et al. Hypofractionated conformal radiotherapy in carcinoma of the prostate: five-year outcome analysis. Int J Radiat Oncol Biol Phys 2003;57:1254–1259.
10. Lukka H, Hayter C, Warde P, et al. A randomised trial comparing two fractionation schedules for patients with localised prostate cancer. Int J Radiat Oncol Biol Phys 2003;57(suppl).

11. Zelefsky MJ, Fuks Z, Hunt M, et al. High dose radiation delivered by intensity modulated conformal radiotherapy improves the outcome of localised prostate cancer. J Urol 2001;166:876–881.

12. Kuban DA, Thames HD, Levy LB, et al. Long- term multi-institutional analysis of stage T1-T2 prostate cancer treated with radiotherapy in the PSA era. Int J Radiat Oncol Biol Phys 2003;57:915–928.

13. Dearnaley DP, Khoo VS, Norman AR, et al. Comparison of radiation side-effects of conformal and conventional radiotherapy in prostate cancer: a randomised trial. Lancet 1999;353:267–272.

14. Pollack A, Zagars GK, Starkschall G, et al. Prostate cancer radiation dose response: results of the M.D. Anderson Phase III randomised trial. Int J Radiat Oncol Biol Phys 2002;53:1097–1105.

15. Ryu JK, Winter K, Michalski JM. Interim report of toxicity from 3D conformal radiation therapy (3D-CRT) for prostate cancer on 3DOG/RTOG 9406, level III (79.2 Gy). Int J Radiat Oncol Biol Phys 2002;54:1036–1046.

16. Zelefsky MJ, Fuks Z, Hunt M, et al. High- dose intensity modulated radiation therapy for prostate cancer: early toxicity and biochemical outcome in 772 patients. Int J Radiat Oncol Biol Phys 2002;53:1111–1116.

17. Kupelian PA, Reddy CA, Carlson TP, et al. Preliminary observations on biochemical relapse-free survival rates after short-course intensity- modulated radiotherapy (70 Gy at 2.5 Gy/fraction) for localised prostate cancer. Int J Radiat Oncol Biol Phys 2002;53:904–912.

18. Roach M III, DeSilvio M, Lawton C, et al. Phase III trial comparing whole-pelvic versus prostate-only radiotherapy and neoadjuvant versus adjuvant combined androgen suppression: Radiation Therapy Oncology Group 9413. J Clin Oncol 2003;21:1904–1911.

19. Nutting CM, Convery DJ, Cosgrove VP, et al. Reduction of small and large bowel irradiation using an optimised intensity-modulated pelvic radiotherapy technique in patients with prostate cancer. Int J Radiat Oncol Biol Phys 2000;48:649–656.

20. Merrick GS, Butler WM, Galbreath RW, et al. Five-year biochemical outcome following permanent interstitial brachytherapy for clinical T1-T3 prostate cancer. Int J Radiat Oncol Biol Phys 2001;51:41–48.

21. Grimm PD, Blasko JC, Sylvester JE, et al. 10-year biochemical (prostate-specific antigen) control of prostate cancer with ^{125}I brachytherapy. Int J Radiat Oncol Biol Phys 2001;51:31–40.

22. Martinez AA, Gustafson G, Gonzalez J, et al. Dose escalation using conformal high-dose-rate brachytherapy improves outcome in unfavourable prostate cancer. Int J Radiat Oncol Biol Phys 2002;53:316–327.

23. Yoshioka Y, Nose T, Yoshida K, et al. High-dose-rate brachytherapy as monotherapy for localised prostate cancer: a retrospective analy-

sis with special focus on tolerance and chronic toxicity. Int J Radiat Oncol Biol Phys 2003;56:213–220.

24. Zelefsky MJ, Leibel SA, Burman CM, et al. Neoadjuvant hormonal therapy improves the therapeutic ratio in patients with bulky prostatic cancer treated with three-dimensional conformal radiation therapy. Int J Radiat Oncol Biol Phys 1994;29:755–761.

25. Henderson A, Langley SEM, Laing RW. Is bicalutamide equivalent to goserelin for prostate volume reduction before radiation therapy? A prospective, observational study. Clin Oncol 2003;15: 318–321.

26. Pilepich MV, Caplan R, Byhardt RW, et al. Phase III trial of androgen suppression using goserelin in unfavourable-prognosis carcinoma of the prostate treated with definitive radiotherapy: report of Radiation Therapy Oncology Group Protocol 85-31. J Clin Oncol 1997;15:1013–1021.

27. Lawton CA, Winter K, Murray K, et al. Updated results of the phase III Radiation Therapy Oncology Group (RTOG) trial 85-31 evaluating the potential benefit of androgen suppression following standard radiation therapy for unfavourable prognosis carcinoma of the prostate. Int J Radiat Oncol Biol Phys 2001;49:937–946.

28. Bolla M, Gonzalez D, Warde P, et al. Improved survival in patients with locally advanced prostate cancer treated with radiotherapy and goserelin. N Engl J Med 1997;337:295–300.

29. Bolla M, Collette L, Blank L, et al. Long-term results with immediate androgen suppression and external irradiation in patients with locally advanced prostate cancer (an EORTC study): a phase III randomised trial. Lancet 2002;360:103–108.

30. Pilepich MV, Winter K, John MJ, et al. Phase III radiation therapy oncology group (RTOG) trial 86-10 of androgen deprivation adjuvant to definitive radiotherapy in locally advanced carcinoma of the prostate. Int J Radiat Oncol Biol Phys 2001;50:1243–1252.

31. Hanks GE, Lu J, Machtay M, et al. RTOG protocol 92-02: a phase III trial of the use of long-term androgen suppression following neoadjuvant hormonal cytoreduction and radiotherapy in locally advanced carcinoma of the prostate. Proc Annu Meet Am Soc Clin Oncol 2000;19:1284.

32. Roach M III, Lu JD, Lawton C, et al. A phase III trial comparing whole-pelvic (WP) to prostate only (PO) radiotherapy and neoadjuvant to adjuvant total androgen suppression (TAS): preliminary analysis of RTOG 9413. Int J Radiat Oncol Biol Phys 2001;51(suppl 1).

33. Roach M III, Lu J, Pilepich MV, et al. Predicting long-term survival, and the need for hormonal therapy: a meta-analysis of RTOG prostate cancer trials. Int J Radiat Oncol Biol Phys 2000;47:617–627.

34. Fellows GJ, Clark PB, Beynon LL, et al. Treatment of advanced localised prostatic cancer by orchidectomy, radiotherapy or combined treatment. A Medical Research Council Study. Urological

Cancer Working Party–Subgroup on Prostatic Cancer. Br J Urol 1992; 70:304–309.
35. Catton C, Gospodarowicz M, Warde P, et al. Adjuvant and salvage radiation therapy after radical prostatectomy for adenocarcinoma of the prostate. Radiother Oncol 2001;59:51–60.
36. Pound CR, Partin AW, Eisenberger MA, et al. Natural history of progression after PSA elevation following radical prostatectomy. JAMA 1999;281:1591–1597.
37. Parker C, Warde P, Catton C. Salvage radiotherapy for PSA failure after radical prostatectomy. Radiother Oncol 2001;61:107–116.

2

Surgical Treatment of Prostate Cancer

Mark R. Feneley and Roger S. Kirby

Key Points

1. Surgery is evolving and new technologies, such as robotics, may offer some patients specific advantages.
2. Surgery may offer patients a survival advantage compared with watchful waiting.
3. Patients with localised poorly differentiated cancers are likely to do better with surgery than radiotherapy.
4. Surgery should be carried out in specialised centres by experienced surgeons.

Introduction

Surgery for prostate cancer has evolved, with the main purpose of curing one of the most common male malignancies at an early stage in its natural history, and preventing the morbidity otherwise associated with unchecked disease progression to more advanced, incurable stages. The operation by which this may be achieved, radical prostatectomy, advanced considerably during the 20th century through developments in anatomical knowledge and surgical experience. It is now a routine surgical procedure in urological oncology carried out through a range of surgical approaches, each with its own advantages and disadvantages.

The first radical prostatectomy operations were done through a perineal approach, adapted from contemporaneous techniques for stone surgery. Theodore Bilroth is credited with the first radical prostatectomy, carried out in 1866; however, the use of this operation was slow to develop owing to its considerable morbidity and mortality. In 1905, Hugh Hampton Young [1] at the Johns Hopkins Hospital, Baltimore, Maryland, described the surgical technique for radical perineal prostatectomy and his results. This was the only definitive treatment available for prostate cancer at that time, preceding Huggins' important work on hormone sensitivity of this disease by 40 years. His technique and its description enabled surgeons to carry out prostatectomy for cure of prostate cancer with substantially lower mortality than previously possible (17%), and a 5-year cure rate of 62% [2]. Incontinence, stricture, fistula, and erectile impotence were nevertheless common and bothersome complications.

Retropubic Prostatectomy

The retropubic approach to radical prostatectomy did not develop until Terence Millin's description of his now classical operation for benign disease, the transcapsular prostatectomy. He adapted this operation to total (radical) prostatectomy, which had not been possible with the transvesical procedures with which surgeons had hitherto become familiar [3]. During the ensuing years, the perineal and retropubic approaches for radical prostatectomy each had its advocates. Radical prostatectomy nevertheless remained a formidable procedure, particularly the retropubic approach, with the risk of uncontrolled hemorrhage from Santorini's plexus. In spite of encouraging cancer-specific outcomes in patients undergoing radical prostatectomy for organ-confined cancer, the surgical difficulties persisted, and rudimentary understanding of surgical anatomy precluded any substantial progress. Complications related, first, to the undocumented course of the periprostatic veins and bleeding consequent to unreliable control, and second, to the unrecognized functional significance of the neurovascular bundles posterolateral to the prostate. Both were described 40 years after Millin's contribution, by Patrick Walsh, at the Johns Hopkins Hospital.

The anatomy of Santorini's plexus and the surgical technique for its control were described by Reiner and Walsh [4] in 1979. This was a landmark contribution, and enabled retropubic radical prostatectomy to be undertaken with a substantially lesser risk of hemorrhage. Surgical control of the dorsal venous complex, and the prospect of a relatively bloodless operative field for the apical dissection of the prostate and urethral preservation were essential steps toward future technical refinements.

Walsh et al.'s [5–7] second pivotal contribution was the anatomical description of the neurovascular bundles and the importance of their formal surgical preservation for postoperative recovery of potency. Walsh et al. showed that the bundles could be separated from the prostate by dissection of the prostatic fascia, along an anterolateral plane, thereby avoiding their injury (by traction or disruption). Applying these two discoveries, Walsh [8] described and subsequently refined the anatomical surgical technique routinely used today. The technique for excision of the neurovascular bundle was described later, along with its indications and impact on outcomes [9].

Perineal Prostatectomy

Retropubic prostatectomy continues to be undertaken with excellent results, though some surgeons prefer the perineal approach. The perineal approach avoids the bleeding sometimes encountered from the dorsal venous complex, as the prostate is removed behind this plane. As a result, the anterior surgical margin can be compromised, and this may have some adverse therapeutic significance in some patients, particularly those with extensive or anterior tumors. Complications specific to this approach relate mostly to anal or rectal injury, with a risk of fecal incontinence, infection, and fistula, but such sequelae are uncommon.

The perineal route does not allow for assessment or removal of pelvic lymph nodes; however, when this is considered important, pelvic lymphadenectomy may need to be carried out as a prior open or laparoscopic procedure. Perineal prostatectomy, therefore, may not be ideal in patients at high risk of a non—organ-confined pathological stage.

Laparoscopic Prostatectomy

Laparoscopic radical prostatectomy has developed within the past 10 years, recognizing the many potential benefits of laparoscopic surgery. It was first described by Schuessler et al. [10] in 1992, and at that time presented significant challenges [11]. Reduction in the extent of surgical incisions, postoperative pain, and analgesic requirement, and shorter convalescence including reduced hospital stay contribute to its potential advantages. Disadvantages relate to the considerable specific skills and experience that need to be acquired and maintained. Procedure-specific advantages and disadvantages must also be considered in relation to open surgery [12].

Operative blood loss in laparoscopic prostatectomy may be minimal by comparison with the open procedure. In experienced hands blood transfusion is rarely required, though this may also apply for the open procedure. For the surgeon, laparoscopy provides an excellent magnified visual field via a monitor, although two-dimensional, and a technological approach to precise operative manipulation. Surgeons undertaking the open procedure may use magnification loupes. The risk of deep vein thrombosis and potentially fatal pulmonary embolism associated with major surgery is always a concern, even with appropriate prophylaxis, and may be increased with prolonged operative times.

Laparoscopic radical prostatectomy became an alternative standard of care to open surgery following the success published by Guillonneau and Vallancien [13] in 2000. Specific advantages, in addition to those generally offered by the laparoscopic approach, arise in the fashioning of the urethrovesical anastomosis. The anastomosis can be made with a continuous suture under direct vision. The magnified field of view allows this to be done with considerable precision, achieving accurate apposition without traction. A watertight anastomosis may minimize potential sequelae of urinary leak and promote functional recovery. Mobilization of the bladder as part of the surgical dissection may also contribute to an apparently more rapid return of urinary continence, and some surgeons have incorporated equivalent maneuvers in the "open" operation for this reason. The urethral catheter can generally be removed at 3 days, and continence appears to be quickly achieved. Overall continence rates appear as good as those achieved by the open procedure. Technical ability and experience substantially influence operative time, which may

may be considerable until substantial experience is gained [14]. Throughout the evolution of today's operation, surgeons have been careful to ensure that the various technical changes introduced would not compromise cancer control. This remains a cornerstone principle in many of the more recent adaptations. The specific challenges of complex laparoscopic surgery have stimulated further advances in surgical technology with the development robotic systems such as AESOP™ (Computer Motion, CA now Intuitive Surgical Corp., Sunnyuale, CA), DaVinca™ (Intuitive Surgical Corp., Sunnyuale, CA) and Zeus™ (Computer Motion, CA, now Intuitive Surgical Corp., Sunnyuale, CA) [15,16]. These systems enable surgeons conventionally trained in open procedures to adapt their skills to use instruments via portals without some of the physical constraints of a laparoscopic environment [14,17,18]. They provide capabilities for precise and remote surgical manipulation, and three-dimensional vision.

Using the robotic approach, extremely favorable early results have been reported from the Vattikuti Institute of Prostatectomy (VIP). Hospital stay is routinely less than 24 hours [19]. Specific modifications incorporated in this form of prostatectomy aim to maximally preserve the cavernosal nerves. The nerves and neurovascular bundles are freed by an anterior dissection of the prostatic fascia, creating on each side a block of tissue referred to as a "veil of Aphrodite." The limited urethral dissection employed may contribute to rapid return of continence, achieved in 90% by 5 months.

Principles of Radical Prostatectomy

Radical prostatectomy is generally carried out with the intent of achieving long-term disease-free survival and thereby cure of early-stage prostate cancer [20]. Secondary, but nevertheless important, concerns are the maintenance of quality of life, in particular continence and erectile function. In some countries, interest is growing in a potentially palliative role in patients with more advanced and noncurable disease. Favorable long-term survival in patients with pathologically organ-confined tumors has been recognized since Young's early experience [21]. In spite of early concerns, nerve sparing does not compromise cure rate [22]. Today, alongside the shift of pathological stage toward organ-confined disease at diagnosis, neurovascular bundles are routinely preserved and bilateral excision is rarely necessary, giving optimal opportunity for maintaining quality of life and functional recovery.

Cancer Control

Cancer-specific outcomes observed after radi- cal prostatectomy have improved substantially within the past 20 years owing to the possibility of detection of earlier stage disease [23]. This is almost entirely attributable to the discovery of prostate-specific antigen (PSA), its increasing availability and clinical use, together with the increasingly prevalent proactive approach toward men's health. Though dependent on patient selection, 10 year biochemical recurrence rates less than 30% can be expected in men with clinically localised cancer, and progression to metastatic disease is rare even without secondary treatment (<10%). Radical prostatectomy is therefore generally not recommended where life expectancy is less than 10 years, particularly in populations exposed to regular PSA testing.

The natural history of prostate cancer following radical prostatectomy is predicted strongly by pathological stage [24]. Although pathological stage can be determined only following surgical treatment, preoperative variables can be combined to provide a useful prediction of pathological stage for individual patients [25]. These variables include clinical stage, serum PSA, and biopsy findings, principally Gleason grade, and each independently correlates with pathological stage. Age also contributes to outcome, and increasing age is associated with less favorable pathological features [26,27]. These pre- and postoperative factors also relate to the risk of metastatic progression following definitive treatment [28].

Wide surgical excision of one neurovascular bundle can sometimes be considered for improved cancer control, and by sparing the contralateral bundle potency may be maintained [9]. Wide excision may be beneficial in a small proportion of cases overall, and rarely necessitates excision of both bundles. Extraprostatic extension frequently occurs at sites additional to the region of the posterolateral bundles, and in this situation contralateral bundle preservation is unlikely to compromise cancer control [29]. In those cases where extraprostatic extension involves the bundle, and negative surgical margins can be achieved by excision, cancer control may be improved [30]. The decision to excise one or both bundles depends on both preoperative and operative findings, including palpable apical tumor on digital rectal examination, perineural invasion, tumor volume, and Gleason score on biopsy, induration of the lateral pelvic fascia at operation, or fixation of the bundles to the prostate [31,32].

In evaluating cancer control following radical prostatectomy undertaken in nonrandomized settings, case selection may impose substantial bias, rendering comparisons of efficacy invalid. Trials of treatment and screening currently being carried out across the world are most important to address ongoing controversies [33,34]. A recently published randomized trial of radical prostatectomy versus watchful waiting for clinically organ-confined cancer showed a significant effect reducing metastatic progression and cancer-specific survival by 8 years (Fig. 2.1) [35]. This study predominantly evaluated treatment of non—PSA-detected tumors; PSA screening undoubtedly increases lead time and thereby also the follow-up required before a treatment-related advantage will be achieved. In spite of the lack of any overall survival difference in this study, the findings imply that the value of

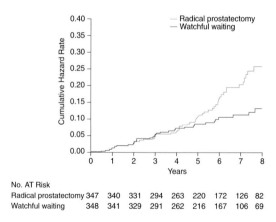

Fig. 2.1. Metastasis—free survival in patients randomized to either radical prostatectomy or watchful waiting [35]. Reproduced with permission from Holmberg L, Bill-Axelson A, Helgesen F, Salo JO, Folmerz P, Haggman M et al. A randomized trial comparing radical prostatectomy with watchful waiting in early prostate cancer. N Engl J Med 2002;347(11):781–789. Copyright © 2002 Massachusetts Medical Society.

curative surgery for early-stage cancer will be acquired with longer follow-up.

Complications

The morbidity of radical prostatectomy today relates principally to erectile dysfunction, but also urinary incontinence. Uncontrolled or unrecognized hemorrhage can be life threatening and can lead to local or systemic complications. Anastomotic stricture can develop in 2% to 20% of patients, and may contribute to difficulties with voiding and urinary control. Rarely, obliteration or distraction at the site of the anastomosis requires more complex procedures and reconstruction. Other significant complications may include infection, lymphatic leak and rarely rectal injury, deep venous thrombosts, and pulmonary embolism.

Erectile Function

In spite of advances in anatomical understanding and surgical technique, bilateral nerve-sparing radical prostatectomy does not assure normal erectile function for all patients. Age, preoperative sexual function, and nerve sparing independently influence the eventual outcome. Sexual inactivity, particularly in the early postoperative period, also may influence the course of functional recovery. Although the return of erectile function may be delayed up to 2 years following surgery, some studies suggest that it may be possible to identify those men unlikely to regain natural erections before that time by nocturnal penile tumescence studies [36]. Tumor stage, race, and patient education have also been implicated [37]. Operative technique, however, is particularly important where other factors are favorable. Rehabilitation using prostaglandin injections and phosphodiesterase type 5 inhibitors may improve outcomes.

Surgical factors that adversely influence early return of sexual activity include perioperative traction or ischemic injury to the cavernous nerves within the posterolateral neurovascular bundles. Visualization and preservation of these nerves during radical prostatectomy may be difficult or imprecise. Their course is indicated by the posterolateral vascular bundles as they are dissected from the prostatic fascia, but the nerves themselves are too small for visualization during surgery, even with a micro-scope. To aid their identification, preoperative electrical stimulation has been evaluated, using the Cavermap™ (Norwood, MA). This device is designed for topographical mapping of erectile responses to electrical stimulation. The impact on subsequent potency, however, has proved unpredictable [38], and in the hands of experienced surgeons negative responses lack specificity [39]. Small variations in surgical technique have been shown to influence potency rates, and a critical review of an intraoperative videotape may identify factors that in the surgeon's hands affect potency [40].

Unilateral excision of the neurovascular bundle adversely influences postoperative potency, but by no means precludes it. As with bilateral nerve sparing, recovery of function after unilateral sparing is influenced by age, and may respond to oral phosphodiesterase inhibitors as neural pathways are at least partially intact. Bilateral excision, however, invariably renders the patient unable to respond to oral phosphodiesterase inhibitors. Reported potency rates with bilateral nerve preservation vary substantially among centers. Many factors may contribute to this observation, perhaps including variation in the reliability with which nerve preservation can be assured at the time of surgery. In those observational studies where unilateral or bilateral excision of the bundles does not adequately correlate with functional recovery, more objective means to ensure and confirm nerve preservation would be invaluable.

A role for sural nerve grafting in late recovery of erectile function, in cases where neurovascular bundle preservation is not feasible, is intriguing and currently being evaluated [41]. Its role in overall surgical management, however, and particularly those cases that involve unilateral bundle excision, remains unproven. Though not a complex additional procedure, nerve grafting does increase operative time and morbidity. Further studies are necessary to determine the contribution of the graft to nerve regeneration after controlling for various factors that may also influence functional recovery.

Urinary Continence

Urinary incontinence following radical prostatectomy is far less common than erectile dysfunction, but when present may have significant implications for the patient. Its true incidence varies according to its definition. Many patients will be continent when the catheter is removed, and among the remainder it may take up to 2 years for continence to be re-established. Occasional patients suffer persistent, troublesome or severe incontinence. For these individuals placement of an artificial urinary sphincter can restore urinary control and quality of life.

Postoperative incontinence generally relates to sphincteric or neurogenic damage acquired during surgery, loss of normal urethral or bladder neck support, periurethral fibrosis, and less frequently detrusor instability. Anastomotic stricture may also need to be excluded. Various techniques for reconstruction or sparing of the bladder neck have been evaluated to improve recovery of continence, mostly without corroborating evidence of any advantage, although some may increase the risk of stricture. Sparing of the neurovascular bundles may itself contribute to preservation of urethral innervation as well as potency, though the principal sphincteric innervation runs with the pudendal nerves. The reported more rapid return of continence following laparoscopic radical prostatectomy would suggest that there may be other technical factors relating to avoidable injury that may contribute to early functional recovery.

Quality of Life

Radical prostatectomy when carried out by experienced surgeons in established centers can maintain excellent quality of life, but such claims may not always be representative in wider surgical practice. The impact of surgery is sudden, recovery may be slow and additional therapy may be required. Changes in sexual function other than potency are inevitable, including changes in perception of orgasm, ejaculation, and libido. The effect of these consequences may vary substantially between individuals.

Outcomes

Outcomes for the retropubic, perineal, and laparoscopic approaches as carried out in the centers of greatest experience are impressive yet extremely difficult to compare. Procedure modifications must be taken into account, such as nerve sparing, which is known to influence outcome, and technical demands specific to the surgical approach, as well as preoperative baseline differences in patients' age, comorbidity, and erectile function [36]. For such reasons, published results based on a surgical series or single centers may not be truly representative of wider outcomes [42–44]. Difficulties in comparing postsurgical morbidity between centers are compounded by the lack of consistency and objectivity in the assessment and definition of continence and potency. Various outcome measures have been used, including physician-reported outcomes, patient-reported outcomes, and neutral data collectors using standardized data collection instruments, which may influence outcome perceptions [43]. Also of concern, factors that determine quality of life and sexual functioning seem to have less than precise relationships with disease and treatment-related morbidity.

Interest has centered on case volume as a factor contributing to outcome following radical prostatectomy, with particular focus on surgeon volume and institution volume. Excellent outcomes have been reported for single-institution, individual surgeon-reported series [13,19, 45–47]. Outcomes reported from high-volume centers suggest lower morbidity and greater consistency; however, favorable outcome does not always follow for high-volume surgeons [48]. Outcomes may be biased by many factors, and those established clinical and operative considerations discussed in previous sections of this chapter should be included for prospectively useful analysis. Individual training and the environment of professional practice may also be significant in influencing outcomes [49]. The importance of operating on a large number of patients to maintain skills and gain experience is widely recognized. Outcomes do vary among individual patients, and although the reliability of auditing this variability relates to case numbers, there may be nonuniformity of institution-, surgeon-, and patient-related factors influencing outcome. For such reasons, valid comparisons are difficult to make, and inevitably the very best outcomes cannot be guaranteed for all patients. Good outcomes, however, can be achieved by appropriately trained and experienced surgeons practicing in institutions of excellence.

Conclusion

Excellent cancer control and quality of life outcomes can be achieved by radical prostatectomy. The key, historical developments emphasize the importance of early diagnosis and consistency in surgical technique. Radical prostatectomy can be carried out by a variety of surgical approaches, and each has advantages and disadvantages. Technological development and application will increasingly influence future surgical practice by improving discrimination of those early-stage tumors that require definitive treatment and more consistently limiting treatment-related morbidity. The results of ongoing randomized controlled trials will add to the evidence base supporting the role of this important treatment option for the many men diagnosed with localized prostate cancer.

Controversies and Outstanding Issues

1. Can we better select patients for surgery on the basis of biological markers?
2. Can we improve imaging techniques to better predict cure following surgery?
3. Can we better standardise clinical practice by centralising surgery and thereby improve surgical outcomes?
4. Can we standardise adjuvant radiotherapy policies?

References

1. Young HH. The early diagnosis and radical cure of carcinoma of the prostate: being a study of 40 cases and presentation of a radical operation which was carried out in four cases. Johns Hopkins Hosp Bull 1905;16:315–321.
2. Young HH, Davis DM. Neoplasms of the urogenital tract. In: Young's Practice of Urology. Philadelphia: WB Saunders, 1926;653–654.
3. Millin T. Retropubic prostatectomy: a new extravesical technique report on 20 cases. Lancet 1945;693–696.
4. Reiner WG, Walsh PC. An anatomical approach to the surgical management of the dorsal vein and Santorini's plexus during radical retropubic surgery. J Urol 1979;121(2):198–200.
5. Walsh PC, Donker PJ. Impotence following radical prostatectomy: insight into etiology and prevention. J Urol 1982;128(3):492–497.
6. Walsh PC, Lepor H, Eggleston JC. Radical prostatectomy with preservation of sexual function: anatomical and pathological considerations. Prostate 1983;4(5):473–485.
7. Lepor H, Gregerman M, Crosby R, Mostofi FK, Walsh PC. Precise localization of the autonomic nerves from the pelvic plexus to the

corpora cavernosa: a detailed anatomical study of the adult male pelvis. J Urol 1985;133:207–212.

8. Walsh PC. Anatomic radical prostatectomy: evolution of the surgical technique. J Urol 1998;160:2418–2424.

9. Walsh PC, Epstein JI, Lowe FC. Potency following radical prostatectomy with wide unilateral excision of the neurovascular bundle. J Urol 1987; 138(4):823–827.

10. Schuessler WW, Kavoussi LR, Clayman RV, Vancaille TH. Laparoscopic radical prostatectomy: initial case report. J Urol 1992; 147(4):246.

11. Schuessler WW, Schulam PG, Clayman RV, Kavoussi LR. Laparoscopic radical prostatectomy: initial short-term experience. Urology 1997;50(6):854–857.

12. Cadeddu JA, Kavoussi LR. Laparoscopic radical prostatectomy: is it feasible and reasonable? Urol Clin North Am 2001;28(3):655–661.

13. Guillonneau B, Vallancien G. Laparoscopic radical prostatectomy: the Montsouris experience. J Urol 2000;163(2):418–422.

14. Bollens R, Roumeguere T, Vanden Bossche M, Quackels T, Zlotta AR, Schulman CC. Comparison of laparoscopic radical prostatectomy techniques. Curr Urol Rep 2002;3(2):148–151.

15. Guillonneau B, Cappele O, Martinez JB, Navarra S, Vallancien G. Robotic assisted, laparoscopic pelvic lymph node dissection in humans. J Urol 2001; 165(4):1078–1081.

16. Abbou CC, Hoznek A, Salomon L, et al. Laparoscopic radical prostatectomy with a remote controlled robot. J Urol 2001;165(6 pt 1): 1964–1966.

17. Prasad SM, Maniar HS, Soper NJ, Damiano RJJ, Klingensmith ME. The effect of robotic assistance on learning curves for basic laparoscopic skills. Am J Surg 2002;183(6):702–707.

18. Stolzenburg JU, Truss MC. Technique of laparoscopic (endoscopic) radical prostatectomy. BJU Int 2003;91(8):749–757.

19. Menon M. Robotic radical retropubic prostatectomy. BJU Int 2003; 91(3):175–176.

20. Han M, Partin AW, Pound CR, Epstein JI, Walsh PC. Long-term biochemical disease-free and cancer-specific survival following anatomic radical retropubic prostatectomy. The 15-year Johns Hopkins experience. Urol Clin North Am 2001;28(3):555–565.

21. Jewett HJ, Bridge RW, Gray GFJ, Shelley WM. The palpable nodule of prostatic cancer. Results 15 years after radical excision. JAMA 1968;203(6):403–406.

22. Walsh PC. Radical prostatectomy, preservation of sexual function, cancer control. The controversy. Urol Clin North Am 1987;14(4): 663–673.

23. Han M, Partin AW, Piantadosi S, Epstein JI, Walsh PC. Era specific biochemical recurrence-free survival following radical prostatec-

tomy for clinically localized prostate cancer. J Urol 2001;166(2): 416–419.

24. Han M, Partin AW, Zahurak M, Piantadosi S, Epstein JI, Walsh PC. Biochemical (prostate specific antigen) recurrence probability following radical prostatectomy for clinically localized prostate cancer. J Urol 2003;169(2):517–523.

25. Partin AW, Mangold LA, Lamm DM, Walsh PC, Epstein JI, Pearson JD. Contemporary update of prostate cancer staging nomograms (Partin Tables) for the new millennium. Urology 2001;58(6):843–848.

26. Khan MA, Han M, Partin AW, Epstein JI, Walsh PC. Long-term cancer control of radical prostatectomy in men younger than 50 years of age: update 2003. Urology 2003;62(1):86–91.

27. Carter HB, Epstein JI, Partin AW. Influence of age and prostate-specific antigen on the chance of curable prostate cancer among men with nonpalpable disease. Urology 1999;53(1):126–130.

28. Pound CR, Partin AW, Eisenberger MA, Chan DW, Pearson JD, Walsh PC. Natural history of progression after PSA elevation following radical prostatectomy. JAMA 1999;281(17):1591–1597.

29. Partin AW, Borland RN, Epstein JI, Brendler CB. Influence of wide excision of the neurovascular bundle(s) on prognosis in men with clinically localized prostate cancer with established capsular penetration. J Urol 1993;150(1):142–146.

30. Smith RC, Partin AW, Epstein JI, Brendler CB. Extended followup of the influence of wide excision of the neurovascular bundle(s) on prognosis in men with clinically localized prostate cancer and extensive capsular perforation. J Urol 1996; 156(2 pt 1):454–457.

31. Shah O, Robbins DA, Melamed J, Lepor H. The New York University nerve sparing algorithm decreases the rate of positive surgical margins following radical retropubic prostatectomy. J Urol 2003; 169(6):2147–2152.

32. Walsh PC. Anatomic radical retropubic prostatectomy. In: Walsh PC, Retik AB, Vaughan ED, Wein AJ, eds. Campbell's Urology. Philadelphia: WB Saunders 2002;3107–3129.

33. de Koning HJ, Auvinen A, Berenguer SA, et al. Large-scale randomized prostate cancer screening trials: program performances in the European Randomized Screening for Prostate Cancer trial and the Prostate, Lung, Colorectal and Ovary Cancer Trial. Int J Cancer 2002;97(2):237–244.

34. Donovan J, Mills N, Smith M, et al. Quality improvement report: Improving design and conduct of randomised trials by embedding them in qualitative research: Protect (prostate testing for cancer and treatment) study. Commentary: presenting unbiased information to patients can be difficult. BMJ 2002;325:766–770.

35. Holmberg L, Bill-Axelson A, Helgesen F, et al. A randomized trial comparing radical prostatectomy with watchful waiting in early prostate cancer. N Engl J Med 2002;347(11):781–789.

36. Stanford JL, Feng Z, Hamilton AS, et al. Urinary and sexual function after radical prostatectomy for clinically localized prostate cancer: the Prostate Cancer Outcomes Study. JAMA 2000;283(3):354–360.

37. Talcott JA, Rieker P, Propert KJ, et al. Patient-reported impotence and incontinence after nerve-sparing radical prostatectomy. J Natl Cancer Inst 1997;89(15):1117–1123.

38. Holzbeierlein J, Peterson M, Smith JA Jr. Variability of results of cavernous nerve stimulation during radical prostatectomy. J Urol 2001;165(1):108–110.

39. Walsh PC, Marschke P, Catalona WJ, et al. Efficacy of first-generation Cavermap to verify location and function of cavernous nerves during radical prostatectomy: a multi-institutional evaluation by experienced surgeons. Urology 2001;57(3):491–494.

40. Walsh PC, Marschke P, Ricker D, Burnett AL. Use of intraoperative video documentation to improve sexual function after radical retropubic prostatectomy. Urology 2000;55(1):62–67.

41. Kim ED, Nath R, Slawin KM, Kadmon D, Miles BJ, Scardino PT. Bilateral nerve grafting during radical retropubic prostatectomy: extended follow-up. Urology 2001;58(6):983–987.

42. Fowler FJ, Roman A, Barry MJ, Wasson J, Lu-Yao G, Wennberg JE. Patient-reported complications and follow-up treatment after radical prostatectomy: the national Medicare experience: 1988–1990 (updated June 1993). Urology 1993;42: 622–629.

43. Talcott JA, Rieker P, Clark JA, et al. Patient-reported symptoms after primary therapy for early prostate cancer: results of a prospective cohort study. J Clin Oncol 1998;16(1):275–283.

44. Heathcote PS, Mactaggart PN, Boston RJ, James AN, Thompson LC, Nicol DL. Health-related quality of life in Australian men remaining disease-free after radical prostatectomy. Med J Aust 1998;168(10): 483–486.

45. Catalona WJ, Carvalhal GF, Mager DE, Smith DS. Potency, continence and complication rates in 1,870 consecutive radical retropubic prostatectomies. J Urol 1999;162(2):433–438.

46. Rabbani F, Stapleton AM, Kattan MW, Wheeler TM, Scardino PT. Factors predicting recovery of erections after radical prostatectomy. J Urol 2000; 164(6):1929–1934.

47. Walsh PC, Marschke P, Ricker D, Burnett AL. Patient-reported urinary continence and sexual function after anatomic radical prostatectomy. Urology 2000;55(1):58–61.

48. Begg CB, Riedel ER, Bach PB, et al. Variations in morbidity after radical prostatectomy. N Engl J Med 2002;346(15):1138–1144.

49. Eastham JA, Kattan MW, Riedel E, et al. Variations among individual surgeons in the rate of positive surgical margins in radical prostatectomy specimens. J Urol 2003;170(6 pt 1):2292–2295.

3

Hormone Therapy for Prostate Cancer

Gairin J. Dancey and Jonathan Waxman

Key Points

1. Combination therapy with an antiandrogen and an LHRH agonist leads to improvement in median survival of 7 months as compared with monotherapy.
2. Intermittent therapy remains a treatment option for patients.
3. Patients with recurrence will respond to further hormonal manipulation.
4. Hormonal therapy has side-effects, some of which can be treated prophylactically.

Introduction

Prostate cancer is now the most prevalent of all male malignancies and the second most common cause of male cancer deaths. Death rates have trebled over the last 30 years, and changes in mortality during this period are shown in Table 3.1 [1].

Prostate cancer is initially an androgen-dependent tumor, and treatment aims to reduce androgen supply to it. It is over a century since the first treatment for prostate cancer was introduced by an English surgeon, who castrated patients with benign and malignant prostatic conditions and observed the responses.

Table 3.1. Prostate cancer mortality

1964	3,370	1965	3,982
1966	3,915	1967	3,903
1968	3,939	1969	4,000
1970	3,906	1971	4,027
1972	4,181	1973	4,236
1974	4,313	1975	4,421
1976	4,611	1977	4,605
1978	4,730	1979	4,837
1980	5,038	1981	5,151
1982	5,291	1983	5,619
1984	6,248	1985	6,628
1986	8,434	1987	7,166
1988	7,458	1989	7,861
1990	8,098	1991	8,570
1992	8,735	1993	8,605
1994	8,689	1995	8,866
1996	8,782	1997	8,531
1998	8,573	1999	8,533
2000	8,293	2001	8,936
2002	8,973		

Source: Office for National Statistics, 2003 [1].

Since that time there have been refinements of treatment so that we are now able to deal more humanely with this condition. We understand more about the toxicities of treatment and the value of second-line therapies. This has led to an improvement in survival. Our hope for the future is that new developments and therapeutic options will result from our increased understanding of the molecular basis of prostate cancer. This chapter surveys the current state of hormonal treatment for prostate cancer.

Localized Disease

The happy triumvirate of watchful waiting, radiotherapy, and surgery are offered patients with localized small-volume prostate cancer. There have been only two randomized trials comparing watchful waiting or radiotherapy with surgery, and they have involved small numbers of patients. In the most recent study, watchful waiting was compared to radical prostatectomy in 695 patients, and there was an increased risk of death in the watch-ful waiting group as compared with the surgical group, with a relative risk of progression to metastatic disease for watchful waiting as compared to surgery of 0.63 (95% confidence interval 0.41–0.96). The advantage to surgery was mostly apparent in those patients with poor prognosis histology [2].

The results of radiotherapy have never been subjected to any significant critical analysis that would stand scrutiny in modern times. Virtually all studies have described results of treatment in single institutions. However, the radiotherapists have managed to climb out of this critical abyss by conducting a significant number of well-organized studies that have examined the role of adjuvant antiandrogen treatment in combination with radiotherapy for localized prostate cancer. In summary, there have been 20 such studies, 14 retrospective and six prospective. Virtually all of the studies have shown an advantage to adjuvant hormonal therapy in terms of the local control of the tumor. However, the situation is distinctly different when one analyzes overall survival. Eighteen of the studies have shown no advantage, and two showed a survival advantage to treatment [3].

The two studies that describe a survival advantage merit further analysis. The first of these studies conducted by the Radiation Therapy Oncology Group (RTOG) is summarized in Table 3.2. In this study there was a significant advantage to patients prescribed adjuvant treatment with goserelin as compared with those patients who received goserelin on progression of their tumor. There are echoes in these results of the 1997 randomized

Table 3.2. Radiotherapy and adjuvant hormonal therapy for localised prostatic cancer: RTOG 8–31

	Goserelin adjuvant	Goserelin on progression	P
Patients	488 (477)	489 (468)	
Nodes + ve	337	345	
Gleason 8–10	139	137	
Local failure	78	135	<0.0001
Distant failure	82	136	<0.0001
Absolute survival	131	138	N.S.

Source: JCO 1997:15;1013.

surgical study in this radiotherapy trial, with the significant improvement in survival confined to those patients with high Gleason grade tumors (Table 3.3). The second study published, in the same year and conducted by the European Organization for Research and Treatment of Cancer (EORTC), randomized patients to radiotherapy with or without 3 years' treatment with goserelin. Kaplan-Meier predictions of 5-year survival showed an improved prospect for those patients treated with adjuvant hormonal therapy [4], and this result was confirmed when the EORTC published in 2000 an update of this trial with actual survival figures (Table 3.4) [5].

Table 3.3. Radiotherapy and adjuvant hormonal therapy for localised prostatic cancer: RTOG 85–31

	Goserelin adjuvant		Goserelin on progression		
	Cancer deaths	Other causes	Cancer deaths	Other causes	P
Gleason 2–7	20	52	22	47	N.S.
Gleason 8–10	25	23	40	20	<0.0001

Source: JCO 1997:15;1013.

Table 3.4. Eortc radiotherapy and adjuvant hormonal therapy trial: the update

Patients:	415 (412)
Median FU:	5.5 yrs
5 year DFS:	40% (95% Cl 32–48%) RT 74% (95% Cl 67–81%) RT + AA
5 year OS:	62% (95% Cl 52–72%) RT 78% (95% Cl 72–84%) RT + AA
5 year disease specific survival:	79% (95% Cl 72–86%) RT 94% (95% Cl 90–98%) RT + AA

Source: Lancet 2002:360;103.

The Hormonal Treatment of Locally Advanced and Metastatic Prostate Cancer

The history of hormonal therapy for prostate cancer dates back to the 1890s, when patients with prostatic diseases, which included cancer, were treated by orchiectomy, and their condition improved. Scientific analyses of the results of treatment emerged nearly a century later, and, after enormous resistance from the urological surgical community, medical therapies for prostate cancer began to replace orchiectomy as a standard treatment for the condition. The urologists argued from the surgical viewpoint that orchiectomy was a simple procedure, and that patients treated in this way could forget about their condition. Medical oncologists argued that it seemed a pretty bad stroke of luck to get cancer, but to be castrated because you had this initial piece of bad luck seemed an unfair twist of fate.

Some 20 years after the initial introduction of the concept of luteinizing hormone–releasing hormone (LHRH) agonist treatment for prostate cancer, treatment with these agents is now accepted as standard. So much so, that the sales of these drugs constituted the biggest oncology earner for big pharmaceutical companies in the late 1990s. These agents are conventionally thought of as acting to downregulate the pituitary gonadal axis. They do this by tight binding to the gonadotropin-releasing hormone (GnRH) receptors in the pituitary. The conformational change resulting from the amino acid substitution leads to greater stability of the molecule, such that the pituitary arymilidases are less able to break down the altered peptide. The result of this is prolonged binding to the receptor and its subsequent downregulation with decreased levels of luteinizing hormone (LH), follicle- stimulating hormone (FSH), and gonadal steroidal hormones. Although this is the convention, it should be noted that there is also a direct effect at the level of the tumor of the GnRH agonists. Hormone-dependent cell lines but not independent lines have higher affinity receptors for these agonists. Both hormone-dependent and -independent cell lines produce GnRH-like peptides, which provide evidence for activity of an autocrine loop in this cancer, and this is confirmed by the presence in human tumors of the GnRH receptor [6].

Combined Antiandrogen Treatment

Labrie, a French Canadian, has made a great contribution to prostate cancer treatment, and suggested that in a disease that is androgen sensitive it is important to eliminate all sources of androgen. Labrie advocated the use of a combination of an antiandrogen with an LHRH agonist in the treatment of prostate cancer. The sources of androgen supplied to the prostate are dietary, adrenal, and testicular. The use of an antiandrogen, such as flutamide, potentially has the benefit of acting synergistically with GnRH agonist. Labrie's early work was not based on any randomized study, and so was not greeted with universal acceptance, but rather the opposite! However, his opinion has been vindicated by randomized controlled trials and meta-analyses of these studies. The randomized trials show a 7-month survival advantage to combination antiandrogen treatment. The meta-analyses, however, do not look at survival advantage, but at overall 5-year survival, and these report a 3% benefit to combination therapy as compared with monotherapy at 5 years. This would appear to be a bizarre time point to use as an assessment, in a disease with a median survival of 3 years. For the clear reason that there is a 7-month survival advantage, it would appear that the appropriate practice recommendation is for combination therapy.

Intermittent Hormonal Therapy

Among the most important quality of life issues for patients with prostate cancer is the loss of sexual function with treatment. For this reason many men delay treatment or take treatment intermittently. There is no evidence whatsoever that intermittent treatment is less successful than continuous therapy. Indeed, if one examines the effects of hormonal treatment on prostate cancer cells growing in culture, then a single exposure to antiandrogen therapy is seen to cause devastating destruction of cell cultures rather akin to the effects of chemotherapy.

There is no rational basis for continuous therapy, and so the intermittent treatment approach can be supported. This point was brought home to me by the clinical course of a patient advocate on one of the trust boards of the Prostate Cancer Charity. He presented with metastatic disease and took hormonal treatment for a period of 6 weeks. He responded well and discontinued treatment until he suddenly presented 4 years later with cord compression, a course of events that might have occurred if he had taken continuous therapy. This anecdote, though hardly hard science, if taken in context and considered in the light of the many side effects of hormonal therapy, could be used to support the case for a randomized trial of intermittent therapy. Certainly this approach is currently more widely advocated and is under investigation [7].

The Treatment of Recurrent Prostate Cancer

There is clinical evidence of prostate-specific antigen (PSA) progression after a median period of 13 months' hormonal therapy. Some 2 years after this evidence emerges, clinical symptoms develop, to be followed a median of 7 months later by death, and this course of events is not what we want for our patients. The biological basis for relapse is of more than passing interest. If patients' biopsy specimens are compared at presentation and relapse, mutations are seen within the androgen receptor in 45% to 55% of patients. It is these mutations that facilitate tumor progression. The androgen receptor is a transcription factor that binds to coactivators and co-repressors together with heat shock proteins, and by this process initiates gene transcription. It may well be that in patients who do not have obvious mutations of the androgen receptor, mutations of coactivators or co- repressors of the androgen receptor are responsible for tumor progression (Fig. 3.1).

These mutations have a practical significance. This significance is that the tumor has changed from being responsive to antiandrogen treatment to becoming dependent on it. In this situation withdrawal of the antiandrogen leads to a transient response, and this is seen in 20% to 40% of patients [8]. Upon further progression, treatment with low-dose steroids leads to a transient response in 10% to 20% of patients. It is very doubtful whether there is any benefit from other agents, such as ketoconazole,

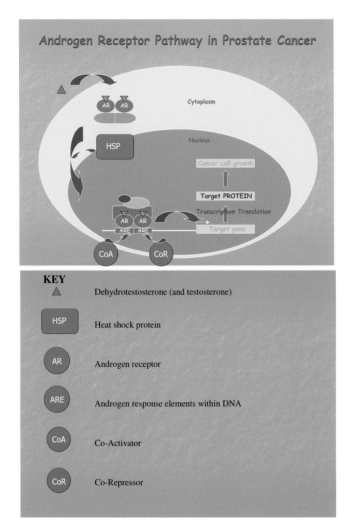

Fig. 3.1. The androgen receptor pathway in prostate cancer. (Courtesy of Dr. Charlotte Bevan, Prostate Cancer Research Group, Department of Cancer Medicine, Faculty of Medicine, Imperial College London, Hammersmith Campus, London, England.)

tamoxifen, or a progestogen. Platelet-derived growth factor receptor (PDGFR) positivity is reported in 10% to 70% of patients' biopsy specimens. For this reason, inhibitors of PDGFR action have been investigated in prostate cancer. Agents inhibiting PDGFR may do so through a number of routes, varying from direct blockade of the receptor itself to inhibition of downstream effector mechanisms. There is no evidence to date that these agents have activity in prostate cancer, though there has been interest recently in the combination of such agents with cytotoxic chemotherapy, and in one such study docetaxel in combination with imatinib has been shown to be of interest [9].

The Side Effects of Hormonal Therapy

In the treatment of any group of patients, there is a historical paradigm to clinical reportage. The initial publication describes an effect of a new treatment. The follow-up publications confirm this effect. A third group of publications then emerge comparing the effect of the new treatment to a standard therapy option, and then finally the side effects of the new treatment are reported. This has been the case with the hormonal treatment of prostate cancer. The initial reports of estrogen activity have been followed by overwhelming evidence of toxicity. This includes a 40% incidence of gastrointestinal toxicity, gynecomastia that is not prevented by the irradiation of breast buds, and cardiovascular toxicity that is not prevented by low-dose anticoagulation [10]. Nevertheless, estrogens are still prescribed in the United Kingdom, although their prescription is proscribed in many other countries in the European Union.

As time has progressed, the GnRH agonists have also been shown to have side effects. These include memory loss, parkinsonism, anemia, and osteoporosis, in addition to the hot flushes and impotence that were obvious from their first use. The most important of the side effects physiologically is osteoporosis, with a loss of bone mass of nearly 10% per annum. Although bisphosphonates have been shown to be of little effect in prostate cancer in terms of limiting pain and tumor progression, which are the main benefits of their use in breast cancer and myeloma, this group of agents is of significant use in limiting osteoporosis in prostate cancer [11].

Conclusion

Over the years the treatment of prostate cancer has certainly become more humane. The most significant area of interest in this disease remains the exploration of the molecular basis for response and relapse. In understanding this, our hope is to provide more effective treatment for prostate cancer.

Controversies and Outstanding Issues

1. Can we extend remission?
2. Can we predict those patients who will benefit from second line therapy on the basis of androgen receptor mutations?
3. Can we limit the side-effects of hormonal therapy, identifying tissue-specific hormonal treatment comparable to the SERMS?

References

1. Office for National Statistics. Mortality Statistics: Cause (Series DH2). HMSO, 2003.
2. Holmberg L, Bill-Axelson A., Helgesen F, et al. A randomized trial comparing radical prostatectomy with watchful waiting in early prostate cancer. N Engl J Med 2002;347:781–789.
3. Pilepich MV, Caplan R, Byhardt RW, et al. Phase III trial of androgen suppression using goserelin in unfavorable-prognosis carcinoma of the prostate treated with definitive radiotherapy: report of Radiation Therapy Oncology Group Protocol 85-31. J Clin Oncol 1997;15:1013–1021.
4. Vicini FA, Kini VR, Spencer W, Diokno A, Martinez AA. The role of androgen deprivation in the definitive management of clinically localized prostate cancer treated with radiation therapy. Int J Radiat Oncol Biol Phys 1999;43:707–713.
5. Bolla M, Collette L, Blank L, et al. Long-term results with immediate androgen suppression and external irradiation in patients with locally advanced prostate cancer (an EORTC study): a phase III randomised trial. Lancet 2002;360:103–106.
6. Qayum A, Gullick W, Clayton RC, Sikora K, Waxman J. The effects of gonadotrophin releasing hormone analogues in prostate cancer are mediated through specific tumour receptors. Br J Cancer 1990; 62:96–99.

7. Goldenberg SL, Bruchovsky N, Gleave ME, Sullivan LD, Akakura K. Intermittent androgen suppression in the treatment of prostate cancer: a preliminary report. Urology 1995;45:839–845.

8. Scher HI, Kelly WK. Flutamide withdrawal syndrome: its impact on clinical trials in hormone-refractory prostate cancer. J Clin Oncol 1993;11:1566–1572.

9. Mathew P, Thall PF, Jones D, et al. Platelet-derived growth factor receptor inhibitor imatinib mesylate and docetaxel: a modular phase I trial in androgen-independent prostate cancer. J Clin Oncol 2004; 22:3323–3329.

10. Bishop MC. Experience with low-dose oestrogen in the treatment of advanced prostate cancer: a personal view. Br J Urol 1996;78:921–927.

11. Dhillon T, Waxman J. Osteoporosis and prostate cancer. Br J Cancer 2003;89:779–780.

4

Chemotherapy in Prostate Cancer

Srikala S. Sridhar and Malcolm J. Moore

Key Points

1. Mitoxantrone and prednisone combination therapy offers symptom palliation but no survival gain.
2. Docetaxel chemotherapy is the first treatment to offer a survival advantage to patients with progressive disease.
3. The use of adjuvant chemotherapy may improved upon the results of hormonal treatment.

Introduction

Prostate cancer is now most frequently diagnosed malignancy and the second leading cause of cancer-related death [1]. Death rates have increased over the past 20 years and mortality may approach that of lung cancer within 15 years [2]. For patients with advanced disease, the response rate to hormonal therapy is about 80%, but this is not durable, and all patients will eventually develop hormone-refractory prostate cancer (HRPC) [3]. Chemotherapy has been shown to have palliative benefit in symptomatic HRPC, but has not yet been demonstrated to prolong survival. Median life expectancy for patients with HRPC is only 12 to 18 months, underscoring the urgent need for new therapeutic approaches [4].

Historically, the role of aggressive systemic chemotherapy in HRPC had been questioned because elderly patients with poor marrow reserve, concomitant illnesses, and poor performance status tolerated it poorly. Coupled with this, chemotherapy trials before 1991 reported response rates of only 5%. In the last decade, the role of chemotherapy in prostate cancer has been revisited, with the development of less toxic regimens, which can significantly improve overall quality of life. Some recent trials in prostate cancer have used quality of life and cancer symptoms as end points. The use of prostate-specific antigen (PSA) has also provided a measure to evaluate the efficacy of newer agents in phase II studies, as most patients with HRPC have disease in bone and do not have conventionally measurable lesions. This chapter discusses the various chemotherapy regimens and recent advances in the systemic management of prostate cancer.

Hormone-Refractory Prostate Cancer

Hormone-refractory prostate cancer is defined as disease that progresses despite castrate testosterone levels, and is refractory to all hormonal manipulations including withdrawal of antiandrogen therapy. Until recently, there had been no standard chemotherapeutic approach for HRPC. Several agents had been evaluated in clinical trials, but many older studies suffered from methodological deficits such as small numbers of patients, heterogeneity of enrolled patients, and lack uniform response criteria [5]. Overall there have been very few recent phase III trials completed in HRPC (Table 4.1) making it difficult to draw firm conclusions about the efficacy of many regimens. However, it would appear that chemotherapy at a minimum does provide a palliative benefit.

Non–chemotherapy-based approaches to palliation also exist. External beam radiotherapy, for example, remains the mainstay of treatment for patients with bone pain, spinal cord compression, or painful urinary obstructive symptoms. In patients with more widespread bone disease, radioisotopes such as strontium-89, rhenium, or samarium may provide some pain relief [6]. Low-dose corticosteroids both with and without chemotherapy are another option for relief of pain and constitutional symptoms [7].

Another class of agents showing palliative benefit in small phase II trials was the bisphosphonates. These are stable

Table 4.1. Summary of recent (1996–2003) phase III trials in hormone refractory prostate cancer (HRPC)

First author, year (reference)	Regimen	No. of patients	>50% PSA decline	Palliative benefit	Time to progression (months)	Overall survival (months)	Median survival (months)
Tannock, 1996 (17)	Mitoxantrone + prednisone vs. prednisone	161	33%* 23%	38% 21%	6.0* 2.5	12.1 11.8	
Kantoff, 1999 (20)	Mitoxantrone + prednisone vs. prednisone	242	38%* 22%		3.7 2.3	12.3 12.6	
Berry, 2002 (21)	Mitoxantrone + prednisone vs. prednisone (asymptomatic)	120	48%* 24%		8.1* 4.1		23 19
Ernst, 2003 (8)	Mitoxantrone + prednisone + clodronate vs. mitoxantrone + prednisone	209	29.7% 28.6%	46% 39%			10.8 11.5
Small, 2000 (53)	Suramin + prednisone vs. prednisone	460	33% 16%	43%* 28%			10.2 10.0
Hudes, 1999 (26)	Vinblastine + estramustine vs. vinblastine	201	25.2% 3.2%		3.7* 2.2		11.9* 9.2

PSA, prostate-specific antigen.
* Statistically significant.

analogues of calcium pyrophosphate that inhibit osteoclast activity in bone, and are approved by the Food and Drug Administration (FDA) for use in the palliation of bone pain due to metastases from breast cancer and myeloma. A phase III trial by Ernst et al. [8], however, failed to demonstrate improvements in palliative response or overall quality of life when the bisphosphonate clodronate, was added to chemotherapy. Similarly, pamidronate, another bisphosphonate, did not significantly palliate bone pain or reduce skeletal-related events (SRE) when compared with placebo [9]. To date, only zoledronic acid, a newer bisphosphonate, appears to significantly reduce SRE and therefore may be a viable option in patients with HRPC [10].

In the past, HRPC patients were identified solely on the basis of symptoms occurring due to increasing tumor burden; but now with the use of the PSA test and imaging studies, patients are often diagnosed with HRPC at a time when they are asymptomatic with a PSA that is starting to rise. The increase in median surviv-al seen in recent HRPC chemotherapy trials when compared with older studies, may thus be less reflective of more effective treatment, but rather represent lead-time bias due to the inclusion of these asymptomatic early-stage patients.

Response to Therapy

One of the more challenging aspects of treating prostate cancer is adequately assessing response to therapy. This is particularly true in the hormone-refractory setting, where disease is often limited to bone, and change in the size or intensity of bone lesions is difficult to interpret. Also, the findings on bone scans may worsen as healing occurs with the initiation of therapy, and may only subsequently slowly improve. Bone scan progression for the purpose of clinical trial entry is now being defined as the appearance of at least one new lesion. Unfortunately, restricting trials to patients with bidimensionally mea-surable soft tissue disease is not a feasible option either, because few patients present this way, and this would exclude otherwise eligible patients.

The PSA, a 34-kd serine protease secreted by both benign and malignant prostate epithelium, is elevated in approximately 95% of patients with advanced metastatic disease, and has been adopted as a surrogate end point in most prostate cancer trials [11]. However, in some settings PSA changes do not show good correlation with firm end points such as survival, leading to the suggestion that the PSA may require validation for the specific clinical setting and therapeutic agent under investigation [12]. There is also no consistent reporting of changes in PSA, making comparisons between trials difficult.

In an attempt to standardize PSA reporting, the PSA working group has created a guideline that defines PSA response as a decline of at least 50% or more, confirmed with a second PSA value at least 4 weeks later (in the absence of clinical or radiographic disease progression). This definition is based on previous studies that suggest a statistically significant survival advantage associated with a PSA decrease of 50% or more [13,14]. Similarly, response duration and time to PSA progression may also be important clinical end points, but have yet to be validated. The PSA is a relatively simple test to obtain, and although it may not be the ideal surrogate marker, it may help to quickly identify those treatments that warrant further investigation at the phase III level.

Measures of response such as PSA do not necessarily indicate whether a patient is benefiting from therapy. Survival and quality of life are the most important measures of patient benefit in the evaluation of treatments in HRPC. Several studies now incorporate palliative end points such as pain, analgesic use, physical activity level, fatigue, appetite, constipation, urinary difficulties, relationships, mood, and overall well-being, through the use of questionnaires such as the Present Pain Intensity (PPI) Index or the Prostate Cancer-Specific Quality of Life Instrument (PROSQOLI). In fact, on the basis of quality of life improvements alone, the chemotherapy regimen of mitoxantrone and prednisone has been approved for use in HRPC.

Mitoxantrone and Prednisone

Mitoxantrone is a synthetic anthraquinone drug that belongs to the anthracenedione class of compounds. It has a symmetrical structure comprising a tricyclic planar chromophore and two basic side chains [15]. The exact mechanism of action of this cell cycle phase nonspecific drug is unclear, but it does appear to (1) intercalate DNA, resulting in inter- and intrastrand crosslinks; (2) bind DNA phosphate backbone, inducing strand breaks; and (3) inhibit topoisomerase II activity. Clinically, mitoxantrone is well tolerated, but due to structural similarity to doxorubicin, it shares the dose-limiting side effect of cardiotoxicity. Other side effects include nausea, vomiting, and myelosuppression [16].

A Canadian study led by Tannock et al. [17] randomized 161 symptomatic patients with HRPC to receive either mitoxantrone every 3 weeks with daily prednisone or prednisone alone. The primary end point of this study was palliative response, which was defined as a significant improvement in either pain or analgesic usage or both (neither could get worse). In the mitoxantrone arm, a statistically significant improvement in pain relief (29% vs. 12%, $p = .01$) and a prolonged duration of this palliative response (43 weeks vs. 18 weeks, $p < .0001$) was demonstrated. These patients also reported improvements in physical and social functioning, global quality of life, anorexia, drowsiness, constipation, and other symptoms [18]. The use of mitoxantrone was also associated with a higher PSA response rate and time to progression. There was no survival benefit of chemotherapy, although a crossover to mitoxantrone in patients who progressed on prednisone was allowed and may have impacted on the survival analysis. An economic analysis of this study by Bloomfield et al. [19] further suggested a benefit to these patients receiving mitoxantrone and prednisone. Overall, these results were consistent with a Cancer and Leukemia Group B (CALGB) study that showed a trend toward greater pain control in the mitoxantrone arm, but no improvement in overall survival (the primary end point). The toxicities of mitoxantrone included neutropenia, thrombocytopenia, and cardiac dysfunction, but in both studies the incidence of serious toxicity was very low [20].

These two critical studies led to FDA approval of mitoxantrone and prednisone for symptomatic patients with HRPC. Its use in earlier stage asymptomatic HRPC patients was recently evaluated in a phase III study by Berry et al. [21], which again suggested no survival benefit. The PSA response in this study (48%) was higher than that seen in the Tannock or CALGB studies (33%), and median survival was also increased to 23 months, as compared to only 12 months in the Canadian and CALGB studies. This may be due to patients having lower median baseline PSA on trial entry, and the lead-time bias introduced by including these early-stage patients.

Estramustine/Taxane-Based Therapy

Estramustine phosphate, a conjugate of estradiol and nitrogen mustard, with hormonal and nonhormonal cytotoxic effects in vitro, has also been evaluated in HRPC [22]. Unlike other alkylating agents, estramustine does not directly damage DNA but depolymerizes cytoplasmic microtubules and microfilaments, binds to microtubule associated proteins, disrupts the nuclear matrix, and inhibits P-glycoprotein [23]. Based on in vitro data suggesting synergy, several phase II studies have been completed using estramustine in combination with etoposide, vinblastine, and the taxanes.

The combination of estramustine and etoposide, which showed in vitro activity, was initially attractive because both drugs target microtubules and could be administered orally. Results from several trials suggest the response rate to be approximately 50%, but this was accompanied by significant toxicity. As a result, this regimen is not in phase III trials [24,25].

Vinblastine, an agent chosen for its distinct antimicrotubule effects, lack of cross-resistance, and nonoverlapping toxicities with estramustine, has also been evaluated. Hudes et al. [26], in a phase III trial, compared estramustine plus vinblastine with vinblastine alone. Response rates in the combined arm were 25.2% versus only 3.2% in the vinblastine alone arm. There was acceptable toxicity, and no survival advantage with the combined arm, but this study was underpowered to detect slight survival improvements. A similar PSA response rate, 24.9%, was reported in a recent study by Albrect et al. [27] for the combination of estramustine and vinblastine. But this was less than the response rate for single-agent estramustine, which was 28.9%. Furthermore, toxicity in the combined arm in this trial was felt to be unacceptable. The difference in tolerability between the trials could be explained by differences in estramustine dosing, or the inclusion of more advanced, poorer performance status patients in the latter trial. Nonetheless, it illustrates the difficulties encountered when testing new agents in HRPC where trial design, drug dosing, and patient selection can play a critical role.

The taxanes (paclitaxel and docetaxel), which also target microtubules, have shown encouraging results when combined with estramustine (Table 4.2). By binding to tubulin, the taxanes induce microtubule stabilization, G2/M phase cell cycle arrest, and apoptosis. They also induce apoptosis through activation of

Table 4.2. Summary of phase II clinical trials of estramustine plus a taxane in patients with hormone-refractory prostate cancer

First author, year (reference)	Regimen	No. of patients	>50% PSA decline	Response in measurable disease	Median survival (months)	1-year survival
Petrylak, 1999 (29)	Docetaxel + estramustine	35	74%	4/7 (57%)	22	77%
Sinibaldi, 2002 (59)	Docetaxel + estramustine	40	45%	3/13 (23%)	N/A	N/A
Savarese, 2001 (60)	Docetaxel + hydrocortisone + estramustine	44	68%	12/24 (50%)	20	
Sitka, 2001 (61)	Docetaxel + estramustine	30	76%	17/30 (57%)		
Hudes, 1997 (22)	Paclitaxel + estramustine	34	53%	4/9 (44.4%)		
Hudes, 2001 (62)	Paclitaxel + estramustine	63	58.1%	6/22 (27.3%)		
Berry, 2001 (31)	Paclitaxel + estramustine	166	48%		15.1	
Athanasiadis, 2003 (63)	Paclitaxel + estramustine	41	58.5%	9/41 (22%)	17	

the proapoptotic protein bax, and inactivation of bcl-2, an anti-apoptotic protein often overexpressed in HRPC. Initial studies with the combination of paclitaxel and estramustine showed activity, but excessive toxicity necessitated dose reductions prior to the phase II trial by Hudes et al. This dose reduction did not compromise antitumor activity, and PSA responses were seen in 53.1% of patients, with a 5.6-month time to progression and a median survival of 17 months [22]. This study also reported a decrease in pain and analgesic requirements, and an improvement in overall quality of life. This combination is now being evaluated in phase III trials.

Despite lowered doses, toxicities due to estramustine, primarily nausea and thromboembolism (requiring prophylactic anticoagulation) continue to be a problem. Berry et al. [28], with the U.S. Oncology Group, conducted a phase II randomized trial comparing estramustine and paclitaxel with paclitaxel alone. Though PSA response rates (48% vs. 25% $p = .01$) and the trend to median survival were higher in the combined arm, there were fewer thromboembolic complications in the paclitaxel only arm, indicating that single-agent paclitaxel may be an option for patients with a history of thromboembolic problems.

Another member of the taxane family that is more potent than paclitaxel and easier from a dosing standpoint is docetaxel. Petrylak et al. [29] treated chemonaive HRPC patients with a combination of estramustine and docetaxel. The PSA responses rates were favorable (74%), but again significant estramustine-related toxicity has led some to question whether single-agent docetaxel is equally effective with less toxicity [29]. A phase II single-agent docetaxel trial by Picus and Schultz [30] showed PSA responses of 45%, with tolerable toxicities. Similarly, Berry et al. [31] reported that in mitoxantrone-pretreated HRPC patients, docetaxel showed a response rate of 41%, with toxicities less than those seen in the estramustine plus docetaxel regimen. Beer et al. [32], using weekly dosing of docetaxel, reported PSA response rate of 47% and pain response of 33%, and the toxicities were all less than 10%. Overall, the positive results with taxane-based therapies have led to its evaluation in several phase III trials (Table 4.3).

Two phase III studies comparing docetaxel-based regimens with mitoxantrone and prednisone have recently been reported. The TAX 327 trial, a prospective, nonblinded, three-arm study, randomized more than 1000 patients to receive docetaxel plus

Table 4.3. Summary of phase II trials using a single-agent taxane in patients with hormone-refractory prostate cancer

First author, year (reference)	Taxane regimen	No. of patients	>50% PSA decline	Response in measurable disease	Time to progression (months)	Survival (months)
Picus, 1999 (30)	Docetaxel 75 mg/m^2 q 3 weeks	35	46%	7/25 (28%)	9	27
Berry, 2001 (31)	Docetaxel 36 mg/m^2/ week ×6 of an 8-week cycle	59	41%	2/6 (33%)	5.1	9.4
Beer, 2001 (32)	Docetaxel 36 mg/m^2/ week ×6 of an 8-week cycle	24	46%	2/5 (40%)	NR	NR
Friedland, 1999 (64)	Docetaxel 75 mg/m^2 q 3 weeks	16	38%	6/9 (67%)	NR	NR
Trivedi, 2000 (65)	Paclitaxel 150 mg/m^2/ week	18	39%	4/8 (50%)	NR	NR

NR, no results.

prednisone (a weekly regimen or every 3 weeks) or the current standard, mitoxantrone and prednisone. End points included overall survival, PSA response, and palliative response. Docetaxel every three weeks led to superior survival (18.9 mo vx. 16.5 mo) and improved rates of response in terms of pain, serum PSA, and quality of life as compared with mitoxantrone plus prednisne [32a]. The Southwest Oncology Group (SWOG) 9916 phase III study randomized 674 patients to receive estramustine and docetaxel or to mitoxantrone and prednisone, with the primary end point being overall survival. The docetaxel and estramustine arm again showed an improvement in overall survival (17.5 mo vs. 15.6 mo) compared with the mitoxantrone arm [32b]. Based on these two large trials, taxane based therapy is quickly becoming the standard of care for hormone refractory prostate cancer.

By combining mitoxantrone, docetaxel, and low-dose prednisone in a phase II multicenter trial, Freeman [33] showed a PSA response rate of 69% and a trend toward improvement in quality of life end points after two cycles of chemotherapy. This is another regimen that will be investigated further.

Triplet Combinations

Triplet combinations of estramustine, paclitaxel, and carboplatin in a small study have shown a 67% PSA response rate but lacked palliative benefit. Other three-drug regimens—estramustine, etoposide, and paclitaxel; paclitaxel, estramustine, and carboplatin; and estramustine, etoposide, and vinorelbine—have shown PSA responses but yet no palliative improvements [34–37]. The value of these three-drug regimens at this time remains largely unknown.

Chemotherapy in Hormone-Sensitive Disease

Neoadjuvant Chemotherapy

The use of systemic chemotherapy earlier in the course of treatment, an effective strategy in some malignancies, has been explored to a small degree in prostate cancer. The objectives of neoadjuvant chemotherapy are to downstage the cancer, decrease the incidence of positive surgical margins, and eliminate micro-metastases. In addition, chemotherapy may eradicate both androgen-independent clones and androgen-sensitive clones, the latter by synergizing with hormonal ablation.

Several pilot neoadjuvant chemotherapy trials have now been reported, and suggest that from a surgical standpoint this is a feasible approach (Table 4.4). Pettaway et al. [38] treated patients with high-risk localized disease with 12 weeks of ketoconazole and doxorubicin alternating with vinblastine and estramustine (KAVE) and androgen ablation followed by radical prostatectomy (RP). The primary end point, a 20% pathological complete response (pCR), was not achieved, but there were fewer positive margins. Clark et al. [39] reported similar results, but increased thromboembolic events, using a neoadjuvant regimen of etoposide and estramustine. The taxanes have also been evaluated in the neoadjuvant setting. Single-agent docetaxel administered prior to RP was well tolerated, with final efficacy results pending at this time [40,41]. Based on encouraging phase II results of the neoadjuvant regimen of docetaxel and estramustine, the CALGB has initiated a phase III randomized study in patients with high-risk disease [42,43]. Other neoadjuvant combinations being studied are docetaxel with mitoxantrone [44], and the CALGB 99811 study of paclitaxel, estramustine, and carboplatin with an luteinizing hormone–releasing hormone (LHRH) agonist.

Administering chemotherapy prior to radical radiation therapy has been studied, but the lack of pathological specimens posttreatment makes interpretation of response somewhat difficult. Zelefsky et al [45] found that neoadjuvant and concomitant estramustine (which may act as a radiosensitizer) and vinblastine with high-dose conformal radiotherapy were well tolerated, but the authors did not draw any conclusions about efficacy. Ben-Josef et al. [46] used a regimen of estramustine and etoposide in patients with high-risk disease preradiotherapy and showed a favorable local control rate (71% vs. 54%) and 5-year disease-free survival (73% vs. 29%) compared with historical controls. In a study by Oh et al. [47], neoadjuvant liposomal doxorubicin chemotherapy prior to androgen ablation plus radiotherapy for high-risk disease showed no activity and significant toxicity.

Although preliminary data suggest that neoadjuvant chemotherapy can be safely administered, larger randomized

Table 4.4. Summary of neoadjuvant chemotherapy trials in prostate cancer

First author, year (reference)	Regimen	Maximum treatment duration (weeks)	Local treatment	No. of patients	+ Margin (%)	Organ confined (%)	Extracapsular extension (%)
Pettaway, 2000 (38)	KAVE + androgen ablation	12	RP	33	17	33	67
Clark, 2001 (39)	Estramustine + etoposide	12	RP	18		31	69
Dreicer, 2001 (40)	Docetaxel	6	RP				
Oh, 2001 (41)	Docetaxel	24	RP				
Hussain, 2003 (42)	Docetaxel + estramustine	18	10 RP 11 RTX RP	21	30		
Eastham, 2003 (43)	Docetaxel + estramustine	18					
Garzotto, 2002 (66)	Docetaxel + mitoxantrone	16	RP	14			
Kelly, 2001 (35)	Paclitaxel + estramustine + carboplatin	16	RTX	56			
Zelefsky, 2000 (45)	Estramustine + vinblastine	24	RTX	27			
Ben-Josef, 2001 (46)	Estramustine + etoposide	6	RTX	18			
Oh, 2003 (47)	Doxil + androgen ablation	8	RTX	7			

KAVE, ketoconazole, doxorubicin, vinblastine, estramustine, RP, radical prostatectomy; RTX, radiotherapy.

controlled trials are necessary to determine its actual benefit. At the present time there is no indication for neoadjuvant chemotherapy outside of a well-designed clinical trial.

Adjuvant Therapy

To date, there are only a few studies published on adjuvant chemotherapy in prostate cancer (Table 4.5). The National Prostate Cancer Project has conducted two randomized trials. Patients postsurgery or post-external beam irradiation were randomized to observation or cyclophosphamide or estramustine. No overall survival benefit in the chemotherapy arm was noticed but an increased progression-free survival was found in patients receiving estramustine [48]. Three additional studies are currently underway. These include the SWOG 9921 phase II study, randomizing post-RP patients to androgen deprivation with Casodex and Zoladex, mitoxantrone and prednisone, or to androgen deprivation alone. RTOG 9902 randomizes patients post–external beam radiotherapy to combined androgen blockade plus four cycles of paclitaxel, etoposide, and estramustine or to combined androgen blockade alone. A third nonrandomized study in high-risk post-RP patients is underway looking at the use of single-agent docetaxel (without androgen ablation).

Targeted Therapies

Our current treatment approaches rely heavily on standard cytotoxic therapies; however, greater insight at the molecular level into cell growth and proliferation has led to the development of targeted biological therapies that offer hope for improved efficacy with minimal toxicity.

Suramin

One of the first biological agents to be studied in prostate cancer was suramin, a polysulfonated aromatic compound initially synthesized as an antiparasitic agent. Suramin was later shown also to interfere with cell signaling, DNA replication, and angiogenesis, and it showed promising cytotoxic activity against prostate cancer cells in vitro [49]. In the clinical setting, patients failing antiandrogen therapy were treated with suramin, which was

Table 4.5. Summary of adjuvant chemotherapy trials in prostate cancer

Author	Adjuvant regimen	Local therapy	Overall survival
National Prostate Cancer Project (48)	Cyclophosphamide + estramustine	Radical prostatectomy, 170 pts; prostate radiotherapy, 233 pts	No benefit
SWOG 9921	Mitoxantrone + prednisone + Casodex + Zoladex	Radical prostatectomy	
RTOG 9902	Paclitaxel + etoposide + estramustine + Casodex + Zoladex	Prostate radiotherapy	
NCI	Docetaxel	Radical prostatectomy	

NCI, National Cancer Institute; pts, patients; RTOG, Radiation Therapy Oncology Group; SWOG, Southwest Oncology Group.

coadministered with a steroid to prevent adrenal suppression. The original clinical trials suggested this was an active compound; however, subsequent studies proved disappointing. Nonetheless, several key lessons were learned during this drug's development.

The importance of antiandrogen withdrawal and steroid use, for example, and the need to control for these confounding variables when designing clinical trials in HRPC, became readily apparent when each of these maneuvers independently demonstrated PSA response rates of 20% to 30%. This likely contributed to the inflated response rates of 70% seen initially in the uncontrolled suramin trials [12]. Another key realization was that PSA was not always a reliable marker of response to therapy as evidenced by trials showing a drop in PSA but no tumor regression or survival benefit, and whether this is a feature common to all biological therapies remains to be determined [12]. Suramin has significant neurological and other side effects owing to its large volume of distribution and long terminal half-life, raising the important issue of appropriate dosing of biological therapies [12]. In summary, the low response rate, lack of survival advantage, and toxicities of suramin have halted its further development, but the lessons learned from this experience can undoubtedly be applied to all future trials of novel therapies in HRPC.

Epidermal Growth Factor Receptor Inhibitors

The epidermal growth factor receptor (EGFR) superfamily of receptors, which comprises four distinct receptors known as EGFR, Human Epidermal growth Factor Receptor, HER2, HER3, and HER4, is a potential therapeutic target in prostate cancer where overexpression is seen in up to 80% of metastasis, and is generally associated with a poorer overall prognosis. Several EGFR targeting agents are now available, including tyrosine kinase inhibitors and monoclonal antibodies. To date, the tyrosine kinase inhibitor gefitinib has undergone the most investigation in prostate cancer. Three phase II trials, with gefitinib alone, and in combination with either docetaxel and estramustine, or mitoxantrone and prednisone, have completed accrual, with final results pending at this time. Two studies, reported in abstract form only, suggest that single-agent gefitinib does not have significant activity [50,51].

Angiogenesis Inhibitors

Targeting angiogenesis is another novel approach. Angiogenesis is a physiological process that is fundamental to cell growth and division. It is initiated by the release of proteases from activated endothelial cells, leading to degradation of the basement membrane, migration of endothelial cells into the interstitial space, and subsequent endothelial proliferation and differentiation into mature blood vessels [52]. Several agents targeting angiogenesis have been tested in prostate cancer, including suramin, thalidomide, matrix metalloproteinase inhibitors, endostatin, angiostatin, vascular endothelial growth factor (VEGF) inhibitors, and cell adhesion inhibitors, to name a few. These are all currently in early stages of development.

Immunotherapy

Another avenue of research in HRPC is immunotherapy, which is dependent on a suitable target antigen being presented to the immune system by an antigen-presenting cell (APC), such as the dendritic cell. The dendritic cell was chosen specifically because it is the most potent in eliciting a T-cell immune response. This approach has been evaluated in a randomized, placebo-controlled, phase III trial in HRPC patients with the drug APC8015. This is a product consisting of autologous dendritic cells loaded ex vivo with a recombinant fusion protein of prostatic acid phosphatase linked to granulocyte-macrophage colony-stimulating factor. This treatment was well tolerated and antigen-specific immunity was evident, but only in the subset of patients with a low Gleason score was there a trend toward improvement in median time to progression. A confirmatory phase III trial in these patients is now underway [53].

Vaccine-based therapies are also being evaluated. In one randomized phase II study, for example, recombinant pox viruses expressing PSA and the b7.1 co-stimulatory molecule were given to patients with nonmetastatic HRPC. Both immunologic activity and a delay in the development of metastatic disease at 6 months was seen [54]. Overall, targeting the immune system provides an exciting and novel approach to treating prostate cancer.

Combinations of Targeted and Cytotoxic Therapy

Targeted therapy in combination with chemotherapy is another area of active research. Several trials have assessed the combination of targeted therapies such as thalidomide, calcitriol, and exisulind with docetaxel. Thalidomide glutarimide is a synthetic glutamic acid derivative that was initially used for morning sickness but was taken off the market due to teratogenicity and neuropathies. Thalidomide has antiangiogenesis effects, inhibits cytokines including tumor necrosis factor-α, and can alter cell adhesion molecules. In a randomized phase II trial with 75 HRPC patients, comparing thalidomide and docetaxel with docetaxel alone, Leonard et al [55] reported a PSA response rate of 50%, and an increase in median survival by 14 months. Gastrointestinal, neurological, and thromboembolic toxicities were reported, the latter necessitating the use of prophylactic anticoagulation. Larger trials incorporating palliative end points, and more data on toxicity are needed to determine whether this combination is a viable option in HRPC.

Another interesting combination is high-dose calcitriol and docetaxel. Calcitriol, at supraphysiological concentrations, is a natural ligand for the vitamin D receptor and its analogues and has several mechanisms of action. Calcitriol causes G0/G1 arrest, changes in p21 (Waf1) and p27 (kip1) expression, dephosphorylation of retinoblastoma protein, downregulation of bcl-2, inhibition of angiogenesis, induction of apoptosis, and changes in several growth factor systems including EGF, transforming growth factor-β (TGF-β), and insulin-like growth factor (IGF). Preclinical studies suggest it enhances cytotoxic activity of docetaxel, paclitaxel, and platinum compounds, and is active in prostate cancer. In the study by Beer [56], HRPC patients treated with oral calcitriol and docetaxel had PSA responses of 81% and tolerated it well. Currently a phase II/III calcitriol study is underway.

Exisulind in an oral agent that selectively induces apoptosis via inhibition of cyclic guanosine monophosphate (cGMP) phosphodiesterase, leading to a sustained increase in cGMP, activation of protein kinase G, and jun kinase, and downstream effects culminating in cell death. Initial clinical studies with exisulind and docetaxel suggest PSA response rates of 44%, but due to toxicities dose reductions are necessary prior to further evaluation [57].

Trials are also currently underway evaluating the drug G3139 with docetaxel. G3139 is an antisense oligonucleotide to bcl-2, an antiapoptotic protein, overexpressed in prostate cancer, and a negative prognostic indicator. This combination has shown PSA responses of 48% and is well tolerated [58]. Other trials using antisense technology are also being initiated.

Taken together, targeted therapies either alone or in combination with chemotherapy are an area of active research that shows promising PSA responses and tolerability.

Summary

Chemotherapy in prostate cancer is an established treatment only for symptomatic hormone-refractory disease, where it can improve symptoms and quality of life but does not impact overall survival. Its role in earlier stage disease is currently being evaluated. Certainly, advancing chemotherapy may eliminate hormone-resistant clones early, thereby slowing the natural progression of this disease. Of the various cytotoxic agents currently under study, the taxanes show the most promise, combining encouraging PSA response rates with tolerability. Targeted therapies both alone or in combination may also prove effective, especially as we gain insight into prostate cancer at the molecular level and learn how best to use these agents. Phase III well-controlled clinical trials of the most promising regimens will then be needed to define the best regimens available.

Controversies and Outstanding Issues

1. Is adjuvant therapy of benefit?
2. Which patient groups will respond to adjuvant chemotherapy?
3. Can we identify patients who will respond to chemotherapy for metastatic disease?
4. Can we produce more effective chemotherapy treatment for patients in relapse?

References

1. Greenlee RT, Hill-Harmon MB, Murray T, Thun M. Cancer statistics, 2001. CA Cancer J Clin 2001;51(1):15–36.

2. Waxman J, Roylance R. New drugs for prostate cancer? Eur J Cancer 1998;34(4):437.

3. Garnick MB. Prostate cancer: screening, diagnosis, and management. Ann Intern Med 1993;118(10):804–818.

4. Ripple GH, Wilding G. Drug development in prostate cancer. Semin Oncol 1999;26(2):217–226.

5. Di Lorenzo G, Autorino R, De Laurentiis M, et al. Is there a standard chemotherapeutic regimen for hormone-refractory prostate cancer? Present and future approaches in the management of the disease. Tumori 2003;89(4):349–360.

6. Porter AT, McEwan AJ, Powe JE, et al. Results of a randomized phase-III trial to evaluate the efficacy of strontium-89 adjuvant to local field external beam irradiation in the management of endocrine resistant metastatic prostate cancer. Int J Radiat Oncol Biol Phys 1993; 25(5):805–813.

7. Moore MJ, Tannock IF. Overview of Canadian trials in hormonally resistant prostate cancer. Semin Oncol 1996;23(6 suppl 14):15–19.

8. Ernst DS, Tannock IF, Winquist EW, et al. Randomized, double-blind, controlled trial of mitoxantrone/prednisone and clodronate versus mitoxantrone/prednisone and placebo in patients with hormone-refractory prostate cancer and pain. J Clin Oncol 2003;21(17): 3335–3342.

9. Small EJ, Smith MR, Seaman JJ, et al. Combined analysis of two multicenter, randomized, placebo-controlled studies of pamidronate disodium for the palliation of bone pain in men with metastatic prostate cancer. J Clin Oncol 2003;21(23):4277–4284.

10. Saad F, Schulman CC. Role of bisphosphonates in prostate cancer. Eur Urol 2004;45(1):26–34.

11. Kelly WK, Scher HI, Mazumdar M, Vlamis V, Schwartz M, Fossa SD. Prostate-specific antigen as a measure of disease outcome in metastatic hormone-refractory prostate cancer. J Clin Oncol 1993; 11(4):607–615.

12. Kaur M, Reed E, Sartor O, et al. Suramin's development: what did we learn? Invest New Drugs 2002;20(2):209–219.

13. Bubley GJ, Carducci M, Dahut W, et al. Eligibility and response guidelines for phase II clinical trials in androgen-independent prostate cancer: recommendations from the Prostate-Specific Antigen Working Group. J Clin Oncol 1999;17(11):3461–3467.

14. Scher HI, Eisenberger M, D'Amico AV, et al. Eligibility and outcomes reporting guidelines for clinical trials for patients in the state of a rising prostate-specific antigen: recommendations from the Prostate-Specific Antigen Working Group. J Clin Oncol 2004; 22(3):537–556.

15. Myers C. Anthracyclines. Cancer Chemother Biol Response Modif 1988;10:33–39.

16. Calabresi P, Chabner BA. Antineoplastic agents. In: Gilman A, Rall TW, Nies AS, eds. Goodman and Gilman's The Pharmacological Basis of Therapeutics. San Francisco: McGraw-Hill, 1993:1241–1244.

17. Tannock IF, Osoba D, Stockler MR, et al. Chemotherapy with mitoxantrone plus prednisone or prednisone alone for symptomatic hormone-resistant prostate cancer: a Canadian randomized trial with palliative end points. J Clin Oncol 1996;14(6):1756–1764.

18. Osoba D, Tannock IF, Ernst DS, et al. Health-related quality of life in men with metastatic prostate cancer treated with prednisone alone or mitoxantrone and prednisone. J Clin Oncol 1999;17(6):1654–1663.

19. Bloomfield DJ, Krahn MD, Neogi T, et al. Economic evaluation of chemotherapy with mitoxantrone plus prednisone for symptomatic hormone- resistant prostate cancer: based on a Canadian randomized trial with palliative end points. J Clin Oncol 1998;16(6): 2272–2279.

20. Kantoff PW, Halabi S, Conaway M, et al. Hydrocortisone with or without mitoxantrone in men with hormone-refractory prostate cancer: results of the cancer and leukemia group B 9182 study. J Clin Oncol 1999;17(8):2506–2513.

21. Berry W, Dakhil S, Modiano M, et al. Phase III study of mitoxantrone plus low dose prednisone versus low dose prednisone alone in patients with asymptomatic hormone refractory prostate cancer. J Urol 2002;168(6):2439–2443.

22. Hudes GR, Nathan F, Khater C, et al. Phase II trial of 96-hour paclitaxel plus oral estramustine phosphate in metastatic hormone-refractory prostate cancer. J Clin Oncol 1997;15(9):3156–3163.

23. Perry CM, McTavish D. Estramustine phosphate sodium. A review of its pharmacodynamic and pharmacokinetic properties, and therapeutic efficacy in prostate cancer. Drugs Aging 1995;7(1):49–74.

24. Pienta KJ, Redman BG, Bandekar R, et al. A phase II trial of oral estramustine and oral etoposide in hormone refractory prostate cancer. Urology 1997;50(3):401–406, discussion 406–407.

25. Dimopoulos MA, Panopoulos C, Bamia C, et al. Oral estramustine and oral etoposide for hormone-refractory prostate cancer. Urology 1997;50(5):754–758.

26. Hudes G, Einhorn L, Ross E, et al. Vinblastine versus vinblastine plus oral estramustine phosphate for patients with hormone-refractory prostate cancer: a Hoosier Oncology Group and Fox Chase Network phase III trial. J Clin Oncol 1999;17(10):3160–3166.

27. Albrecht W, Van Poppel H, Horenblas S, et al. Randomized Phase II trial assessing estramustine and vinblastine combination chemotherapy vs estramustine alone in patients with progressive hormone-escaped metastatic prostate cancer. Br J Cancer 2004; 90(1):100–105.

28. Berry WG, Dakhil M, Hathorn S, et al. Phase II randomized trial of weekly paclitaxel (Taxol®) with or without estramustine phosphate in

patients with symptomatic, hormone-refractory, metastatic carcinoma of the prostate (HRMCP). Proc Am Soc Clin Oncol 2001;20:696(abstract 175a).

29. Petrylak DP, Macarthur R, O'Connor J, et al. Phase I/II studies of docetaxel (Taxotere) combined with estramustine in men with hormone-refractory prostate cancer. Semin Oncol 1999;26(5 suppl 17):28–33.

30. Picus J, Schultz M. Docetaxel (Taxotere) as monotherapy in the treatment of hormone-refractory prostate cancer: preliminary results. Semin Oncol 1999;26(5 suppl 17):14–18.

31. Berry W, Dakhil S, Gregurich MA, et al. Phase II trial of single-agent weekly docetaxel in hormone-refractory, symptomatic, metastatic carcinoma of the prostate. Semin Oncol 2001;28(4 suppl 15):8–15.

32. Beer TM, Pierce WC, Lowe BA, et al. Phase II study of weekly docetaxel in symptomatic androgen-independent prostate cancer. Ann Oncol 2001;12(9):1273–1279.

32a. Tannock IF, de Wit R, Berry WR, et al. Docetaxel plus prednisone or mitoxantrone plus prednisone for advanced prostate cancer. N Engl J Med 2004;351:1502–1512.

32b. Petrylak DP, Tangen CM, Hussain MHA, et al. Docetaxel and Estramustine compared with mitoxantrone and prednisone for advanced refractory prostate cancer. N Engl J Med 2004;351:1513–1520.

33. Freeman S. A phase II study of the combination of docetaxel/mitoxantrone/low-dose prednisone in men with hormone refractory cancer (HRPC). Proc Am Soc Oncol 2003;22:432(abstract 1735).

34. Colleoni M, Graiff C, Vicario G, et al. Phase II study of estramustine, oral etoposide, and vinorelbine in hormone-refractory prostate cancer. Am J Clin Oncol 1997;20(4):383–386.

35. Kelly WK, Curley T, Slovin S, et al. Paclitaxel, estramustine phosphate, and carboplatin in patients with advanced prostate cancer. J Clin Oncol 2001;19(1):44–53.

36. Smith DC, Esper P, Strawderman M, et al. Phase II trial of oral estramustine, oral etoposide, and intravenous paclitaxel in hormone-refractory prostate cancer. J Clin Oncol 1999;17(6):1664–1671.

37. Gilligan T, Kantoff PW. Chemotherapy for prostate cancer. Urology 2002;60(3 suppl 1):94–100, discussion 100.

38. Pettaway CA, Pisters LL, Troncoso P, et al. Neoadjuvant chemotherapy and hormonal therapy followed by radical prostatectomy: feasibility and preliminary results. J Clin Oncol 2000;18(5):1050–1057.

39. Clark PE, Peereboom DM, Dreicer R, et al. Phase II trial of neoadjuvant estramustine and etoposide plus radical prostatectomy for locally advanced prostate cancer. Urology 2001;57(2):281–285.

40. Dreicer R, Klein EA. Preliminary observations of single-agent docetaxel as neoadjuvant therapy for locally advanced prostate cancer. Semin Oncol 2001;28(4 suppl 15):45–48.

41. Oh WK, George DJ, Kaufman DS, et al. Neoadjuvant docetaxel followed by radical prostatectomy in patients with high-risk localized prostate cancer: a preliminary report. Semin Oncol 2001;28(4 suppl 15):40–44.
42. Hussain M, Smith DC, El-Rayes BF, et al. Neoadjuvant docetaxel and estramustine chemotherapy in high-risk/locally advanced prostate cancer. Urology 2003;61(4):774–780.
43. Eastham JA, Kelly WK, Grossfeld GD, et al. Cancer and Leukemia Group B (CALGB) 90203: a randomized phase 3 study of radical prostatectomy alone versus estramustine and docetaxel before radical prostatectomy for patients with high-risk localized disease. Urology 2003;62(suppl 1):55–62.
44. Beer TM, Garzotto M, Lowe BA, et al. Phase I study of weekly mitoxantrone and docetaxel before prostatectomy in patients with high-risk localized prostate cancer. Clin Cancer Res 2004;10(4):1306–1311.
45. Zelefsky MJ, Kelly WK, Scher HI, et al. Results of a phase II study using estramustine phos- phate and vinblastine in combination with high-dose three-dimensional conformal radiotherapy for patients with locally advanced prostate cancer. J Clin Oncol 2000;18(9):1936–1941.
46. Ben-Josef E, Porter AT, Han S, et al. Neoadjuvant estramustine and etoposide followed by concurrent estramustine and definitive radiotherapy for locally advanced prostate cancer: feasibility and preliminary results. Int J Radiat Oncol Biol Phys 2001;49(3):699–703.
47. Oh WK, Kaplan ID, Febbo P, et al. Neoadjuvant doxil chemotherapy prior to androgen ablation plus radiotherapy for high-risk localized prostate cancer: feasibility and toxicity. Am J Clin Oncol 2003;26(3):312–316.
48. Schmidt JD, Gibbons RP, Murphy GP, et al. Adjuvant therapy for clinical localized prostate cancer treated with surgery or irradiation. Eur Urol 1996;29(4):425–433.
49. Takano S, Gately S, Neville ME, et al. Suramin, an anticancer and angiosuppressive agent, inhibits endothelial cell binding of basic fibroblast growth factor, migration, proliferation, and induction of urokinase-type plasminogen activator. Cancer Res 1994;54(10):2654–2660.
50. Moore MJ, Winquist E, Pollak M, et al. Randomized phase II study of two doses of gefitinib ("Iressa," ZD1839) in hormone-refractory prostate cancer: a trial of the National Cancer Institute of Canada-Clinical Trials Group. Ann Oncol 2002;13(suppl 5):90.
51. Rosenthal MT, Gurney GC, Davis H, et al. Inhibition of the epidermal growth factor receptor (EGFR) in hormone refractory prostate cancer (HRPC): initial results of a phase II trial of gefitinib. Proc Am Soc Clin Oncol 2003;22:416 (abstract 1671).

52. Sridhar SS, Shepherd FA. Targeting angiogenesis: a review of angiogenesis inhibitors in the treatment of lung cancer. Lung Cancer 2003;42(suppl 1):S81–91.
53. Small EJ, Fratesi P, Reese DM, et al. Immunotherapy of hormone-refractory prostate cancer with antigen-loaded dendritic cells. J Clin Oncol 2000; 18(23):3894–3903.
54. Arlen PM, Gulley JL, Tsang KY, Schlom J. Strategies for the development of PSA-based vaccines for the treatment of advanced prostate cancer. Expert Rev Vaccines 2003;2(4):483–493.
55. Leonard GDD, Gulley WL, Arlen JL, Figg PM. Docetaxel and thalidomide as a treatment option for androgen-independent, nonmetastatic prostate cancer. Rev Urol 2003;5(suppl 3):S65–70.
56. Beer TM. Development of weekly high-dose calcitriol based therapy for prostate cancer. Urol Oncol 2003;21(5):399–405.
57. Pruitt-Scott DE, Ryan CW, Stadler WM, et al. Exisulind (EXI) plus docetaxel (DOC) for hormone-refractory prostate cancer (HRPC). Proc Am Soc Clin Oncol 2002;21:161b(abstract 2460).
58. Chi K, Murray RN, Gleave ME, et al. A phase II study of oblimersen sodium (G3139) and docetaxel (D) in patients (pts) with metastatic hormone-refractory prostate cancer. Proc Am Soc Clin Oncol 2003; 22:393(abstract 1580).
59. Sinibaldi VJ, Carducci MA, Moore-Cooper S, Laufer M, Zahurak M, Eisenberger MA. Phase II evaluation of docetaxel plus one-day oral estramustine phosphate in the treatment of patients with androgen independent prostate carcinoma. Cancer 2002;94(5):1457–1465.
60. Savarese DM, Halabi S, Hars V, et al. Phase II study of docetaxel, estramustine, and low-dose hydrocortisone in men with hormone-refractory prostate cancer: a final report of CALGB 9780. Cancer and Leukemia Group B. J Clin Oncol 2001;19(9):2509–2516.
61. Sitka Copur M, Ledakis P, Lynch J, et al. Weekly docetaxel and estramustine in patients with hormone-refractory prostate cancer. Semin Oncol 2001;28(4 suppl 15):16–21.
62. Hudes GRM, Conroy J, Habermann J, Wilding T. Phase II study of weekly paclitaxel (P) by 1-hour infusion plus reduced-dose oral estramustine (EMP) in metastatic hormone-refractory prostate carcinoma (HRPC): a trial of the Eastern Cooperative Oncology Group. Proc Am Soc Clin Oncol 2001;20:175a(abstract 697).
63. Athanasiadis A, Tsavdaridis D, Rigatos SK, Athanasiadis I, Pergantas N, Stathopoulos GP. Hormone refractory advanced prostate cancer treated with estramustine and paclitaxel combination. Anticancer Res 2003;23(3C):3085–3088.
64. Friedland D, Cohen J, Miller R Jr, et al. A phase II trial of docetaxel (Taxotere) in hormone-refractory prostate cancer: correlation of antitumor effect to phosphorylation of Bcl-2. Semin Oncol 1999;26 (5 suppl 17):19–23.

65. Trivedi C, Redman B, Flaherty LE, et al. Weekly 1-hour infusion of paclitaxel. Clinical feasibility and efficacy in patients with hormone-refractory prostate carcinoma. Cancer 2000;89(2):431–436.
66. Garzotto M, Higano C, Lowe B, et al. Neoadjuvant weekly docetaxel and mitoxantrone in patients with high risk localized prostate cancer: a phase I trial. Proc Am Soc Clin Oncol 2002;21:155b (abstract 2434).

5

Treatment Options in Superficial (pTa/pT1/CIS) Bladder Cancer

Jeremy L. Ockrim and Paul D. Abel

Key Points

1. There are substantial differences in recurrence and progression rates denoted by prognostic factors.
2. Intravesical adjuvant therapy reduces local recurrence.
3. BCG is likely to be the best adjuvant intravesical agent.
4. A case can be made for maintenance therapy with BCG.
5. There is no good evidence that BCG improves overall survival.

Introduction

Bladder cancer is the fourth most common cancer in men and the eighth most common cancer in women worldwide, and the incidence continues to rise. In the United Kingdom, 13,600 new cases per annum contribute 5% to the national cancer burden [1]. Over 100,000 diagnostic, check, and interventional cystoscopies each year are performed in surveillance protocols in attempting to monitor for disease progression. In the United States, there were approximately 57,500 new cases and 12,500 deaths in 2003, resulting in an annual expenditure ($2.2 billion/year) almost twice that for prostate cancer [2]. These figures reflect the lifelong commitment to surveillance and intervention for recurrent and progressive disease. The difficulties involved in this complex process were emphasized in McFarlane et al.'s [3] seminar in 1996, where considerable divergence of opinion was noted among clinicians presented with a variety of clinical scenarios. This chapter provides an overview of the current rationale behind the therapeutic options available for superficial bladder cancer treatment. In this way, it is hoped to empower clinicians with a broad sweep of the evidence on which therapy is based.

Current Issues in Superficial Bladder Cancer Classification

The current system of bladder tumor classification is based on the International Union Against Cancer (UICC) revision of 1997 [4]. *Superficial bladder cancer* is the term used to describe transitional cell carcinomas with histopathological categories pTa and pT1 as well as carcinoma in situ (CIS); pTa tumors are confined to the urothelium bordered by the basement membrane, whereas pT1 tumors have penetrated into the lamina propria. Much debate has been concerned with the inclusion of pT1 tumors as "superficial," with an implication of indolent natural history. In fact, the depth of penetration into and beyond the lamina propria may be the single most important prognostic factor for "superficial" bladder cancers [5,6] (both vascular and lymphatic invasion have also been suggested as important prognostic factors [7,8]). As such, subcategorization of pT1 tumors has been proposed, dividing pT1 tumors into "up to muscularis mucosae" (pT1a), "into muscularis mucosae" (pT1b), and "beyond muscularis mucosae" (pT1c) [8,9]. The dependence of the urologist on the uropathologist is fundamental to this classification. Concern persists that even experienced uropathologists may vary in their interpretation of tissue, not only among themselves, but also with themselves over time [10]. One study has demonstrated that pathologists often overstage but undergrade bladder specimens [11]. The importance of good-quality resection specimens, including the underlying detrusor muscle (see Role of Transurethral Resection and Tumor Surveillance, below) and of good liaison between urologist and uropathologist (which ideally should be centralized within a multidisciplinary setting) is clear.

Natural History of Superficial Bladder Cancer and Prognostic Factors

Because the type and timing of adjuvant therapy for superficial bladder cancer depends on the prediction of biological change from an indolent to an aggressive phenotype, a good understanding of the natural history of the disease is essential for the working practice of urologists and oncologists. Because even patients with low-grade, low-stage superficial bladder cancers are now subjected to adjuvant therapy, contemporary data of untreated tumors are sparse. This is of particular relevance to high-risk tumor groups, where it is now unacceptable for modern trials to contain an "untreated" arm. As a result, outcomes have to be compared to historical data. All analyses and any conclusions from data must be assessed with this limitation in mind.

Grade

Many series have shown the importance of tumor grade in rates of recurrence and progression. The National Bladder Cancer Collaborative Group (NBCCG) trial [12] reported progression rates for World Health Organization tumor grades I, II, and III of 2%, 11%, and 45%, respectively, figures reflected in many similar studies [5,13].

Stage

Between 70% and 80% of new bladder tumors are superficial on presentation: 70% pTa and 30% pT1 [14]. Despite the presumption that bladder cancer develops through a logical sequence of biological events from superficial to invasive disease, pTa and pT1 tumors show substantial differences in their potential to progress to muscle invasion. Several series have shown that progression is nearly always associated with pT1 disease. The NBCCG demonstrated that progression occurs in only 3% of pTa tumors, compared with 30% of pT1 tumors [12]. The risk of progression is closely correlated with mortality. The 5-year mortality rate for pTa tumors is less than 1%, whereas the 5-year mortality for pT1 tumors is as high as 24% [5,15]. As such,

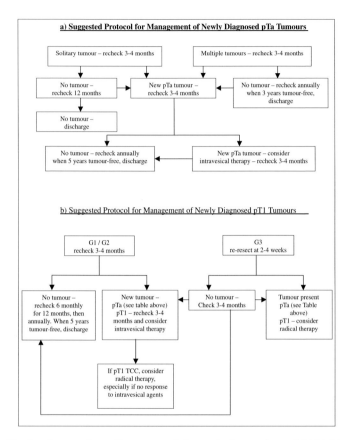

Fig. 5.1. Suggested surveillance protocols for newly diagnosed superficial bladder cancers. (From Abel PD. Follow-up of patients wih a "superficial" transitional cell carcinoma of the bladder: the case for a change in policy. Br J Urol 1993;72(2):135–142, Blackwell Publishing Ltd.)

separate protocols for pTa and pT1 cystoscopic surveillance have been proposed [15] (Fig. 5.1).

Frequency of Recurrence

The intervals between tumor recurrences are of central importance. Recurrence rates steadily decrease with the length of disease-free interval, such that the risk of further disease is less than 10% after 5 years of negative cystoscopic examination [16,17]. Fitzpatrick et al. [18] demonstrated that the first check cystoscopy also pointed to future tumor activity; 80% of those with a clear 3-month cystoscopy remained disease free, whereas those with recurrent disease at 3 months had only a 10% chance of remaining disease free in the 2 years thereafter. The European Organization for the Research and Treatment of Cancer–Genitourinary Group (EORTC-GU) also reviewed the importance of initial treatment failure as a prognostic factor for long-term outcome [16]. The overall recurrence rate following transurethral tumor ablation was approximately 50% to 70%. This rate was substantially affected by the early clinical response; over 75% of those with rapidly recurrent lesions developed subsequent recurrences. It is important to recognize that early tumor recurrence may also be related to surgical technique (see Role of Transurethral Resection and Tumor Surveillance, below).

Multifocality and Tumor Size

Multicentric presentation and tumor volume are also important prognostic factors. At diagnosis, 30% of lesions are multiple [17], and these carry a poorer prognosis than solitary tumors, with shorter disease-free intervals and higher progression rates [19,20]. Tumor sizes greater than 3 cm and 5 cm have also been correlated with poorer outcome [12,20].

Carcinoma in Situ (CIS)

Carcinoma in situ is defined as a flat (nonpapillary) high-grade transitional cell carcinoma that has not penetrated the basement membrane of the epithelium. Such lesions are considered distinct entities from papillary (pTa/pT1) tumors, with profound implications for prognosis. Clinically, CIS can be divided into diffuse (velvety erythematous elevations) or focal (thickened white metaplasia) lesions. Diffuse CIS is nearly always reflected in filling (storage) bladder symptoms and positive urine cytology, whereas focal CIS is frequently a marker for subsequent papillary tumor development. These two subsets of CIS have marked differences in invasive potential. In Lamm's [21] review, an overall progression rate of 54% was reported for untreated CIS.

Riddle et al. [22] showed muscle invasion occurring in 58% of those with diffuse disease, compared with only 8% of those with focal urothelial (CIS) abnormalities. Association with papillary tumors increases the risk. The series reported by Althausen et al. [23] and Herr et al. [24] showed progression rates of 83% and 71% when CIS and papillary tumor were noted together. Moreover, with diffuse CIS, occult disease of the distal ureters and prostatic urethra may be present in as many as 60% [25]. In cases of suspected (diffuse) CIS, sampling of the prostatic urethra is essential, especially as positive biopsies would preclude orthotopic bladder reconstruction.

Relative Risk of Clinical Prognostic Factors

The factors that predict the biological potential of superficial lesions must be correctly weighted before deciding on cystoscopic surveillance protocols and adjuvant therapy. The relative importance of the prognostic factors was measured by multivariate analyses of two Medical Research Council (MRC) trials [26] and two EORTC-GU trials [20]. In the MRC analyses, tumor number at presentation and tumor recurrence at the first followup cystoscopy at 3 months were statistically better at predicting recurrence than all other prognostic factors. The confidence of these observations compared with the (subjective) interpretation of other histopathological data led Hall et al. [27] to propose a cystoscopic and adjuvant chemotherapy protocol based on these two factors alone. In the EORTC-GU analyses, the relative risk of disease progression was assessed [20]. The greatest risk was in those with frequent disease recurrence, followed by tumor grade and size. Surprisingly, the T stage at presentation (pTa/pT1) did not add to the prognostic calculation. The authors proposed stratification of superficial bladder tumors into three different prognostic (risk) groups on which clinicians may decide the necessity of adjuvant therapy (Table 5.1). Although these tables are interesting research tools, most clinicians assess risk according to all the available clinical and histological information (Table 5.2), applied on an individual basis, and according to the needs of the patient.

Table 5.1. Risk index for patients in various subgroups

Recurrence rate (per year) Tumor size (cm)	<1			1 to 3			>3		
	<1.5	1.5–3	>3	<1.5	1.5–3	>3	<1.5	1.5–3	>3
G1	1	1	1	1	2	2	2	2	3
G2	1	2	2	2	2	3	3	3	3
G3	2	2	2	2	3	3	3	3	3

Note: Each cell gives the risk index pertaining to progression and disease-specific mortality. Risk index estimated from the Cox model including only three factors: tumor size, G grade, and recurrence rate. The estimated Cox models for progression is 0.51 recurrence rate + 0.84 G grade + 0.48 tumor size, and for death is 0.89 recurrence rate + 0.73 G grade + 0.44 tumor size. Adapted from Kurth et al. [20].

Table 5.2. Suggested prognostic factors influencing management of superficial bladder tumors

Low risk (conservative management)	High risk (surgical management*)
No involvement of muscularis mucosae (<pT1b)	Involvement into or beyond the muscularis mucosae (pT1b and pT1c)
Small (less than 1.5 cm)	Large (greater than 1.5 cm) tumor
Solitary tumor	Multifocal tumors
Absence of associated carcinoma in situ	Presence of carcinoma in situ (especially if distant to papillary tumor site)
Second endoscopic resection showing no residual tumor (at 3 months)	Second endoscopic resection showing residual tumor (at 3 months)
Good response to intravesical chemotherapy/ immunotherapy	Poor response to intravesical chemotherapy/immunotherapy
No tumor recurrence during the first year of surveillance cystoscopy	Early recurrence less than 6 months after initial resection

* Surgical management (cystectomy/cystoprostatectomy) for high-grade, high-stage (G3pT1) disease.

Molecular Markers

The search to find alternate prognostic factors on which to base treatment decisions (conservative versus radical intervention for high-risk tumors) has shifted to the molecular level. Many markers have been proposed, including altered expression of *p53*, *p21*, *Ki-67*, *bcl-2*, *EGFR*, *c-erb B2*, cyclooxygenase-2 (COX-2), and E-cadherin [28]. Of these, the most studied is the *p53* tumor-suppressor gene. Overexpression of *p53* is correlated with stage and grade, and in some studies has been linked to an increased risk of disease progression [29]. Unfortunately, a recent meta-analysis [30] of 138 publications on the predictive value of *p53*, including nearly 4000 patients, failed to find to any significant correlation that could be applied in daily clinical practice. Moreover, *p53* expression has not been useful in predicting response to adjuvant (bacille Calmette-Guerin [BCG]) therapy [29]. As yet, the potential of molecular makers remains unfulfilled.

Role of Transurethral Resection (TUR) and Tumor Surveillance (Recurrence and New Occurrence)

Cystoscopic visualization of the bladder remains the primary modality of diagnosis, surveillance, and treatment of superficial bladder tumors. Attention to and accurate documentation of the relevant clinical prognostic factors are essential components for future therapeutic decisions. This should include estimation of tumor number, size, position, and configuration as well as the intervals between recurrences. Tissue sampling by TUR is advocated from all the affected areas to document the worst stage and tumor grade, and the presence of muscle in the biopsy specimen is essential to allow the uropathologist to accurately stage the tumor (see Natural History of Superficial Bladder Cancer and Prognostic Factors, above). Routine (random) biopsies of macroscopically normal urothelium to identify dysplasia are not useful, as less than 10% of normal-appearing urothelium in either pTa or pT1 disease will show an abnormality [31]. Moreover, significant variations in the interpretation of histological samples may in fact hinder rather than benefit therapeutic decisions [32].

It was previously assumed that the incidence of recurrence is low following cystoscopic extirpation of tumor, and that most treatment failure is a result of new occurrences in remote areas of de novo urothelial dysplasia. It is now apparent that as many as 50% of recurrences are due to tumor reimplantation at the time of original resection, as evidenced by molecular studies that demonstrate that many synchronous and metachronous lesions are of similar clonal origin [33,34]. Early tumor recurrences, which are multifocal and orientated toward the bladder dome (which occur in less than 5% of first presentations), are more likely to be as a result of the mechanical dispersion of "freed" tumor cells during resection (which gravitate upward) rather than genuine new occurrences. Later recurrences are more likely to be of disparate clonal derivation and represent genuine new occurrences. It is interesting to note that it is only the incidence of early tumor recurrence that is reduced by intravesical chemotherapy; the rate of later recurrences is unchanged (see Intravesical Therapy and Dose Scheduling, below) [35].

It is accepted that conventional light cystoscopy is an insensitive method of visualizing all superficial tumors and areas of subtle urothelial abnormality. Up to one third of tumors may be missed using conventional light sources, and inadequate resection is commonplace [36]. In one series of pT1 disease [37], recurrent tumor was detected in 43% of those subjected to repeat resection of the original resection site, emphasizing the importance of second look cystoscopy, re-resection, and early (3-month) surveillance. This is particularly relevant for high-risk tumors. Several series have demonstrated that up to 30% of these tumors are upstaged to muscle-invasive disease with a second resection [38]. Recent attempts to overcome the limitations of conventional white light cystoscopy, using the protoporphyrin 5-aminolevulinic acid (ALA) and blue light, have been reported to enhance visualization and direct tumor ablation [39]. Rates of local recurrence may also be reduced using laser ablation, which may be exploited to more precisely ablate lesions (and less likely to disperse cells) than the standard TUR diathermy loop [40]. These techniques have been successful in reducing recurrence rates by up to 15% in small, uncontrolled series [39,40]. Although these methods have considerable development ahead, they highlight the importance of scrupulous TUR technique to all operating clinicians.

Role of Intravesical Therapy in Tumor Prophylaxis

The purpose of intravesical adjuvant therapy is threefold: to eradicate residual tumor, to reduce the rate of recurrence, and to reduce the risk of tumor progression. Many different topical instillation agents have been proposed and tried over three decades. However, only two classes of cytotoxic agent and one immunotherapeutic modulator have been established with (limited) clinical efficacy, and are in common use. These are the anthracycline antibiotics Adriamycin and epirubicin, the alkylating agents thiotepa and mitomycin C (MMC), and the mycobacterium bacille Calmette-Guerin (BCG).

Intravesical Chemotherapy and Recurrence/Progression Rates

Intravesical chemotherapy agents were traditionally adminis-tered as delayed bladder instillations initiated at least 1 week fol-lowing transurethral resection of the tumor and continued for up to 6 weeks. Such regimes were originally intended as prophylaxis against new occurrences, and had been demonstrated in many series to effect significant reductions in the short-term tumor recurrence rates. Early recurrence rates (within 1 year) for low-grade (G1 or G2), low-stage (pTa) superficial tumors can be reduced by up to 33% using anthracyclines [41] and 33% to 50% using MMC [42], although these rates are adversely affected by increasing tumor stage and grade [43]. Unfortunately, good initial responses have proven less durable with prolonged tumor sur-veillance. In a review of 2861 patients enrolled in controlled studies up to 1992 [42], the long-term reduction in tumor recur-rence averaged only 17%. Indeed, in those followed 5 years or more, the recurrence rate increased to that achieved using transurethral extirpation alone [44]. Neither has this figure improved significantly by protracted maintenance therapy [45,46]. The cumulative data from such studies suggests that the overall reduction in recurrence rates using intravesical chemotherapy is approximately 12% to 15% [47]. Even more dis-appointing is the failure of chemotherapy to affect overall progression rates. The EORTC-GU/MRC meta-analysis demon-strated that intravesical chemotherapy has no impact on either stage progression or overall survival [48]. No study to date has demonstrated a significant improvement in these parameters using chemotherapy agents.

Intravesical Immunotherapy and Recurrence/Progression Rates

Intravesical immunotherapy using BCG was first proposed by Morales et al. [49] in 1976. Conventional prophylactic regimes of 6 weekly instillations, similar to those used for chemotherapy, resulted in complete response rates of 60% to 100% at 1 year, 55% to 75% after 2 years, and mean recurrence-free intervals of 10 to

22.5 months [50]. Although the long-term response rates with BCG are less enduring, the reduction in recurrence appears to be better than the rates achieved using most chemotherapy agents. This superiority is supported by comparative studies of BCG and anthracycline agents, which suggest that BCG has a roughly twofold advantage over Adriamycin and epirubicin (with an overall BCG tumor recurrence rate reduction of approximately 30%) [51]. In contrast, trials comparing MMC directly with BCG have been less consistent in outcome, and passionately debated. Of the published comparative MMC-BCG studies, three have suggested that MMC may have therapeutic equivalence to BCG for patients with low risk stage pTa and lower grade 1 and 2 tumors [52–54]. The inter- and cross-trial inconsistencies (inclusion criteria) and the interpretation of clinical and pathological factors have compounded the problems of analyses. However, in each of these three studies, the BCG schedules used were suboptimal. The balance of evidence still suggests an (small) advantage for BCG immunotherapy. Series reported by the Finnbladder Group [55] and Lundholm et al. [56] showed short-term response rates between 49% and 65% for BCG, compared with 34% and 38% for MMC. The Southwest Oncology Group (SWOG) trial 8795 was terminated early when a significant advantage for high-risk patients was demonstrated for those in the BCG arm [57]. In a recent meta-analysis of published and unpublished MMC-BCG comparative studies, seven of the 11 trials demonstrated superiority for BCG with mean 2-year recurrence rates of 46.4% and 38.6%, respectively [58]. It must be recognized that it has not yet been established whether this advantage is durable. The current American Urological Association (AUA) guidelines (published in 1999) still recommend the use of either MMC or BCG for the prophylaxis of pT1 and high-grade pTa disease [59].

Despite many studies, definitive evidence that BCG immunotherapy improves the overall survival for those with superficial bladder cancer has not been established. However, BCG may affect the rate of disease progression. Some of the largest studies that have attempted to assess the risk of progression are shown in Table 5.3. These studies can be criticized for their inclusion criteria, power (most having an insufficient number of patients to detect small differences in outcome) and ill-defined end points. Accepting these limitations, there now exists a body of evidence that suggests that BCG therapy may delay stage progression or delay the necessity for radical

Table 5.3. Selected studies of disease progression following bacille Calmette-Guérin (BCG) immunotherapy

Study (year)	Study design	No. of patients	Follow-up (months)	Progression*
Herr (86) (1988)	TUR alone vs. BCG induction	86	72	37% TUR vs. 28% BCG ($p = .01$)
Martinez-Pineiro (87) (1990)	BCG induction vs. thiotepa induction and maintenance monthly (year) vs. Adriamycin induction and maintenance monthly (year)	176	36	1.5% BCG vs. 3.6% thiotepa vs. 7.5% Adriamycin
Lamm (88) (1991)	BCG induction and maintenance 6 monthly (2 years) vs. Adriamycin induction and monthly maintenance (year)	131	65	6% BCG vs. 16% Adriamycin (not significant)
Pagano (89) (1991)	TUR alone vs. BCG induction and maintenance monthly (year) and quarterly (second year)	126	21	17% TUR vs. 4% BCG ($p < .05$)
Lamm (69) (2000)	BCG induction vs. BCG induction and six monthly maintenance (3 years)	384	60	30% induction vs. 24% maintenance ($p = .04$)
Millan-Rodriguez (90) (2000)	Retrospective analysis of TUR alone vs. BCG vs. chemotherapy	1529	50	Relative risk of progression decreased 0.3 for BCG
Sylvester (60) (2002)	Meta-analysis of 24 trials	4863	30	9.8% BCG vs. 13.8% controls ($p = .001$)

TUR, transurethral resection.
* The wide variation in progression rates reflects the widely different inclusion criteria and definitions of disease progression used in different studies.

(cystectomy or radiotherapy) intervention for those with high-risk disease. This view is supported by Sylvester et al.'s [60] meta-analysis of 4863 patients enrolled in 24 trials (see Treatment Options in G3pT1 Disease, below) [60].

Intravesical Therapy and Dose Scheduling

The traditional induction regimen of six weekly instillations of chemotherapy, initiated a week after resection, was based on original work using BCG immunotherapy. Delayed bladder instillation was intended as a *prophylactic* therapy for a secondary new occurrence, presuming that all previous tumors have been eradicated. It is now increasingly apparent that intravesical chemotherapy is best intended as an *ablative* therapy to "mop up" loose cells released at the time of extirpation and to prevent tumor reimplantation. Longitudinal studies have shown that tumor recurrences occur in two time-dependent peaks. The groups with early recurrence peaks are sensitive to chemotherapy, whereas those with delayed recurrences are generally resistant [35]. It is not surprising, therefore, that the influential study of the MRC demonstrated that immediate instillation of MMC within 24 hours of transurethral resection was as effective as conventional 6-week courses [61]. Indeed, more recent studies have suggested that intravesical chemotherapy should be administered as soon after resection as possible, with most of the advantage being lost within the first 24 hours [62]. Immediate bladder instillation appears to be safe as long as there is no risk of perforation and the bleeding has been adequately controlled. For those with extensive resection, the risk of systemic absorption and side effects should be considered. Cutaneous reactions often involving the genitalia and palms have been noted in up to 9% of patients receiving MMC [63]. BCG immunotherapy should never be given in the perioperative setting, as this increases the risk of systemic absorption and infection.

The optimal BCG treatment schedule remains a matter of some debate. A second 6-week cycle of BCG therapy improves the overall response rate from 50% to 70% [64], and 30% to 50% of those who fail an initial course of BCG respond to a second 6-week induction course [64,65]. As a result, many trials have attempted to improve BCG efficacy using "maintenance" regimens of continued weekly, biweekly, or monthly instillations [66], as well as longer induction courses [67]. Although one review of 14 such trials [68] suggested that response rates were maximized with additional BCG courses and led to a more durable long-term advantage over single-induction regimens, only one randomized study has proven any (statistically significant) advantage for progression. The SWOG 8507 study [69] showed a disease-free improvement from 40% to 61% and a 6% reduction in the rate of surgical intervention in patients receiving 3-week maintenance instillations at 3 and 6 months and every 6 months thereafter over 3 years. However, only 16% of the 243 patients were able to tolerate the complete 3-year regimen due to the local side effects. Overall, only a third to one half of the patients in these studies were able to tolerate regular BCG instillations due to the cumulative BCG-induced cystitis [68,69]. The toxicity of maintenance regimes (consisting of up to 27 instillations over a 3-year period) has also been addressed by the EORTC-GU group. The analysis of their own and other studies [19,70,71] suggests that the toxicity is mostly incurred during the induction phase, and lowering the dose of the maintenance (one-third dose) could reduce the limiting toxicity to 20%. It remains to be seen if the EORTC results can be translated into the common experience of most urology practices. For most, the therapeutic advantages of maintenance regimes are compromised by significant increases in local toxicity.

Role of Bacille Calmette-Guérin in the Treatment of Carcinoma in Situ

To date, BCG remains the treatment of choice for CIS disease. Although cytotoxic chemotherapy agents have shown initial response rates as good as 48% using anthracyclines and 53% for MMC, most series have demonstrated that this response is time limited, with fewer than 20% remaining disease free at 5 years [72]. This apparent chemoresistance may well reflect the high grade of CIS disease, whereas higher grade may imply greater antigenicity and therefore susceptibility to BCG immunotherapy. Bacille Calmette-Guerin therapy gives complete response rates of 60% to 70% with a median duration beyond 3 years and projected 5-year responses of 45%. Nevertheless, 30% to 40% of patients with CIS disease do not respond to a single induction course of

BCG [72]. The response rates and the durability of response may be improved with maintenance therapy. Advocates of long-term maintenance refer to the SWOG 8507 study (see above) [69], although this was not specific for CIS. Further credence to maintenance BCG therapy has been offered by the more recent meta-analysis of Sylvester et al. [60]. Of the 403 patients with CIS disease treated with maintenance regimens, the relative advantage over no therapy was 35% and the overall risk of progression was 13.9% after 2.5 years. If patients are committed to repeated BCG courses, judicious monitoring for disease recurrence and progression (including extravesical sites) is paramount. Each consecutive induction course following CIS recurrence has a diminishing therapeutic value and an increased risk of disease progression. Current European Association of Urologists (EAU) guidelines recommend a second course for patients who fail primary therapy, and consideration of radical intervention (cystectomy) thereafter [73].

Treatment Options in G3pT1 Disease

G3pT1 forms the watershed of therapeutic intervention, with advocates of conservative and radical intervention equally persuaded in their differing interpretation of the available data. The historical series suggest that untreated G3pT1 has a recurrence rate between 70% and 80%, and progression rates ranging from 29% to as high as 50% [74]. In Birch and Harland's [75] review, 40% of G3pT1 cases followed beyond 24 months developed muscle-invasive disease. Although it is now accepted that treatment with transurethral resection for G3pT1 disease alone is inadequate, it is also apparent that a significant proportion of G3pT1 patients do not experience disease progression, and for these patients (early) cystectomy would represent an overtreatment. The challenge remains to find a way of identifying and reducing the risk of progression while safely conserving the bladder.

The decision to opt for conservative (bladder-sparing) treatment obligates the use of adjuvant BCG immunotherapy, despite an acceptance that the impact of BCG therapy on G3pT1 tumors has been difficult to assess. This is due in part to the limited number of patients with G3pT1 disease available for study (who will accept enrollment in a study arm with no adjuvant therapy),

but also to the interdependence of other factors such as concomitant CIS, tumor multifocality, tumor size, and previous
recurrence rates. The nonstandardization of BCG treatment protocols has also limited direct comparisons of data. Historical
reports of response rates following BCG therapy have varied from
25% to 75% for recurrence and 7% to 54% for progression
[76–78]. Important differences would account for the large
variation in responses. For example, in Herr's [76] 1991 series,
where progression rates were high (54%) all the selected patients
had multiple tumor recurrences. In contrast, in Cookson and
Sarosdy's [77] study, in which post-BCG progression rates
were significantly lower (19%), only 30% of the patients had
had a prior recurrence. In Serretta et al.'s [78] series, patients
were treated with various chemotherapy and combination
regimens; all the patients with poor (clinical) prognostic indicators of response were excluded, resulting in progression rates of
only 12%. The lack of a randomized control throws open
the question of whether this apparent success was due to
the chemotherapy or the patient selection process. Some of
the more recent series using BCG therapies alone are summarized
on Table 5.4.

Although the numbers of patients enrolled in studies with
"unpolluted" G3pT1 disease are limited, clinicians are obliged to
take guidance from the evidence base as a whole. The recent
meta-analysis of Sylvester et al. [60] of all superficial bladder
cancers enrolled in randomized studies of BCG therapy suggests
a 27% reduction in the odds of progression, but only for those
receiving maintenance protocols over a period of 3 years. There
was no statistically significant benefit for either overall or
disease-specific survival, raising the question of the durability of
the benefit beyond 3 years. For those who received only single or
a duplicate course of BCG the progression rate was similar to that
of resection alone. From the accumulation of such data has
emerged a "rule of threes," in which a third of those with G3pT1
disease treated by BCG survive with their bladder in situ, a third
survive after cystectomy, and a third die from their disease
despite all interventions [10]. Although cystectomy can result in
recurrence free rates as good as 78% at 10 years [79], those who
advocate a conservative policy argue that such results simply
reflect the natural history of the disease. Nevertheless, the preservation of the bladder in situ, even as a temporized objective, could
be considered a worthwhile benefit to some patients.

Table 5.4. Recent studies of BCG immunotherapy for G3pT1 disease

Study (year)	Study design	No. of patients	Follow-up (years)	Result
Cookson (91) (1997)	BCG (one or more induction)	48	15	Progression 35% within 5 years, 16% 5–10 years, 10% 10–15 years
Pansadoro (92) (2002)	BCG (induction and maintenance)	81	6.3	Recurrence 33%; progression 15%
Patard (93) (2002)	TUR alone or delayed BCG and BCG primary induction	80	5	Progression TUR alone or delayed BCG 53% vs. BCG primary induction 36%
Shahin (10) (2003)	TUR alone and BCG (one or more induction)	153	5.3	Recurrence TUR alone 75% vs. BCG 70%; progression TUR alone 36% vs. BCG 33%

Other Immunomodulators

The relative success of BCG has stimulated interest in other immunomodulators for use as adjuvant intravesical agents. Interferons (IFNs) are key components of the cytokine response, causing increased expression of major histocompatibility complex antigens on transitional cells, activating T cells, lymphokine activated killer cells, and natural killer cells. Intravesical IFN-α2b has demonstrated the most activity against bladder cancer. Several small studies have now been reported [80–82]. These early data have shown moderate tumor responses (recurrence rates reduced by approximately 15%), although the responses and the relapse rates are inferior to those for BCG and MMC [81,82]. Although it is likely that BCG (as well as MMC) as monotherapy is superior, in vitro studies have suggested that the combination of IFN-α and standard intravesical agents may have a synergistic effect [82]. Pilot studies have already shown a synergistic action of IFN-α with epirubicin [83], MMC [84], and BCG [85], whereas the combination of BCG and IFN-α effected a 55% secondary response in 40 patients who were prior BCG failures [51]. The numbers in these preliminary studies have all been small and the follow-up limited. Further large-scale trials are awaited before interferon therapy is more widely adopted.

Conclusion

Many patients with bladder cancer are elderly, with extended comorbidity, and a careful ap-proach to their treatment is necessary. Atten-tion to and accurate documentation of relevant clinical and histopathological prognostic factors allows stratification into low-, intermediate-, and high-risk groups. Diffuse carcinoma in situ is considered a separate and aggressive disease cat-egory. The timing of future surveillance cys-toscopy and interventional adjuvant therapy are dependent on these criteria. A change in risk classification should prompt a reevaluation of patient status.

In all patients, the initial approach is to attempt cystoscopic tumor ablation. Adjuvant intravesical therapy is decided by the prognostic status and the dynamic of stage change. For those with low- or intermediate-risk lesions, cytotoxic chemotherapy immediately following resection is the first choice. High-risk lesions including G3pT1 disease and CIS should be treated with intra-vesical BCG immunotherapy. Maintenance regimens may confer a reduction in progressive potential but at a cost of increased risk of toxicity. Concomitant poor prognostic factors or failure of BCG therapy (reappearance of tumor or positive urine cytology) is an indi-cation for more aggressive therapy. In these patients radical cystectomy is indicated.

The role of alternative immunomodulators, combination and dose-modulated instillation protocols, and molecular prognosti-cators is promising, although their potential is dependent on further large-scale study.

Controversies and Outstanding Issues

1. Can we identify biological markers for response to BCG?
2. Can we develop new agents for the treatment of superficial bladder cancer?
3. Can we identify agents that are better tolerated than BCG?
4. Can we identify molecular markers which predict the natural history in an individual patient?

References

1. Office of National Statistics. Cancer trends Table 3.1: Bladder cancer, key statistics. www.statistics. gov.uk/StatBase/xsdataset.asp.
2. Jemal A, Tiwari RC, Murray T, et al. Cancer statistics, 2004. CA Cancer J Clin 2004;54(1):8–29.
3. McFarlane JP, Ellis BW, Harland SJ. The management of superficial bladder cancer: an interactive seminar. Br J Urol 1996;78(3):372–378.
4. International Union Against Cancer. Urinary Bladder. In: Sobin LH, Wittekind Ch, eds. TNM Classification of Malignant Tumours. New York: Wiley-Liss, 1997:187–190.
5. Anderstrom C, Johansson S, Nilsson S. The significance of lamina propria invasion on the prognosis of patients with bladder tumors. J Urol 1980;124(1):23–26.
6. Abel PD, Hall RR, Williams G. Should pT1 transitional cell cancers of the bladder still be classified as superficial? Br J Urol 1988; 62(3):235–239.
7. Lopez JI, Angulo JC. The prognostic significance of vascular invasion in stage T1 bladder cancer. Histopathology 1995;27(1):27–33.
8. Smits G, Schaafsma E, Kiemeney L, Caris C, Debruyne F, Witjes JA. Microstaging of pT1 transitional cell carcinoma of the bladder:

identification of subgroups with distinct risks of progression. Urology 1998;52(6):1009–1013.

9. Angulo JC, Lopez JI, Grignon DJ, Sanchez-Chapado M. Muscularis mucosa differentiates two populations with different prognosis in stage T1 bladder cancer. Urology 1995;45(1):47–53.

10. Shahin O, Thalmann GN, Rentsch C, Mazzucchelli L, Studer UE. A retrospective analysis of 153 patients treated with or without intravesical bacillus Calmette-Guerin for primary stage T1 grade 3 bladder cancer: recurrence, progression and survival. J Urol 2003; 169(1):96–100.

11. Witjes JA, Kiemeney LA, Schaafsma HE, Debruyne FM. The influence of review pathology on study outcome of a randomized multicentre superficial bladder cancer trial. Members of the Dutch South East Cooperative Urological Group. Br J Urol 1994;73(2):172–176.

12. Heney NM, Ahmed S, Flanagan MJ, et al. Superficial bladder cancer: progression and recurrence. J Urol 1983;130(6):1083–1086.

13. Malmstrom PU, Busch C, Norlen BJ. Recurrence, progression and survival in bladder cancer. A retrospective analysis of 232 patients with greater than or equal to 5-year follow-up. Scand J Urol Nephrol 1987;21(3):185–195.

14. Donat SM. Evaluation and follow-up strategies for superficial bladder cancer. Urol Clin North Am 2003;30(4):765–776.

15. Abel PD. Follow-up of patients with "superficial" transitional cell carcinoma of the bladder: the case for a change in policy. Br J Urol 1993;72(2):135–142.

16. Brausi M, Collette L, Kurth KH, et al. Variablity in the recurrence rate at first follow-up cystoscopy after TUR in stage TaT1 transitional cell carcinoma of the bladder: a combined analysis of seven EORTC studies. Eur Urol 2002;41(5):523–531.

17. Heney NM, Proppe K, Prout GR Jr, Griffin PP, Shipley WU. Invasive bladder cancer: tumor configuration, lymphatic invasion and survival. J Urol 1983;130(5):895–897.

18. Fitzpatrick JM, West AB, Butler MR, Lane V, O'Flynn JD. Superficial bladder tumors (stage pTa, grades 1 and 2): the importance of recurrence pattern following initial resection. J Urol 1986;135(5):920–922.

19. Dalesio O, Schulman CC, Sylvester R, et al. Prognostic factors in superficial bladder tumors. A study of the European Organization for Research on Treatment of Cancer: Genitourinary Tract Cancer Cooperative Group. J Urol 1983;129(4):730–733.

20. Kurth KH, Denis L, Bouffioux C, et al. Factors affecting recurrence and progression in superficial bladder tumours. Eur J Cancer 1995; 31A(11):1840–1846.

21. Lamm DL. Carcinoma in situ. Urol Clin North Am 1992;19(3): 499–508.

22. Riddle PR, Chisholm GD, Trott PA, Pugh RC. Flat carcinoma in Situ of bladder. Br J Urol 1975;47(7):829–833.

23. Althausen AF, Prout GR Jr, Daly JJ. Non-invasive papillary carcinoma of the bladder associated with carcinoma in situ. J Urol 1976;116(5): 575–580.

24. Herr HW, Wartinger DD, Fair WR, Oettgen HF. Bacillus Calmette-Guerin therapy for superficial bladder cancer: a 10–year followup. J Urol 1992;147(4):1020–1023.

25. Utz DC, Farrow GM. Carcinoma in situ of the urinary tract. Urol Clin North Am 1984;11(4):735–740.

26. Parmar MK, Freedman LS, Hargreave TB, Tolley DA. Prognostic factors for recurrence and followup policies in the treatment of superficial bladder cancer: report from the British Medical Research Council Subgroup on Superficial Bladder Cancer (Urological Cancer Working Party). J Urol 1989;142(2 pt 1):284–288.

27. Hall RR, Parmar MK, Richards AB, Smith PH. Proposal for changes in cystoscopic follow up of patients with bladder cancer and adjuvant intravesical chemotherapy. BMJ 1994;308(6923):257–260.

28. Soloway MS, Sofer M, Vaidya A. Contemporary management of stage T1 transitional cell carcinoma of the bladder. J Urol 2002;167(4): 1573–1583.

29. Smith ND, Rubenstein JN, Eggener SE, Kozlowski JM. The p53 tumor suppressor gene and nuclear protein: basic science review and relevance in the management of bladder cancer. J Urol 2003;169(4): 1219–1228.

30. Schmitz-Drager BJ, Goebell PJ, Ebert T, Fradet Y. p53 immunohistochemistry as a prognostic marker in bladder cancer. Playground for urology scientists? Eur Urol 2000;38(6):691–699.

31. van der Meijden AP, Oosterlinck W, Brausi M, Kurth KH, Sylvester R, de Balincourt C. Significance of bladder biopsies in Ta,T1 bladder tumors: a report from the EORTC Genito-Urinary Tract Cancer Cooperative Group. EORTC-GU Group Superficial Bladder Committee. Eur Urol 1999;35(4):267–271.

32. Richards B, Parmar MK, Anderson CK, et al. Interpretation of biopsies of "normal" urothelium in patients with superficial bladder cancer. MRC Superficial Bladder Cancer Sub Group. Br J Urol 1991; 67(4):369–375.

33. Sidransky D, Frost P, Von Eschenbach A, Oyasu R, Preisinger AC, Vogelstein B. Clonal origin bladder cancer. N Engl J Med 1992; 326(11):737–740.

34. Takahashi T, Habuchi T, Kakehi Y, et al. Clonal and chronological genetic analysis of multifocal cancers of the bladder and upper urinary tract. Cancer Res 1998;58(24):5835–5841.

35. Hinotsu S, Akaza H, Ohashi Y, Kotake T. Intravesical chemotherapy for maximum prophylaxis of new early phase superficial bladder carcinoma treated by transurethral resection: a combined analysis of trials by the Japanese Urological Cancer Research Group using smoothed hazard function. Cancer 1999;86(9):1818–1826.

36. Zaak D, Kriegmair M, Stepp H, et al. Endoscopic detection of transitional cell carcinoma with 5-aminolevulinic acid: results of 1012 fluorescence endoscopies. Urology 2001;57(4):690–694.

37. Klan R, Loy V, Huland H. Residual tumor discovered in routine second transurethral resection in patients with stage T1 transitional cell carcinoma of the bladder. J Urol 1991;146(2):316–318.

38. Herr HW. The value of a second transurethral resection in evaluating patients with bladder tumors. J Urol 1999;162(1):74–76.

39. Filbeck T, Pichlmeier U, Knuechel R, Wieland WF, Roessler W. Clinically relevant improvement of recurrence-free survival with 5-aminolevulinic acid induced fluorescence diagnosis in patients with superficial bladder tumors. J Urol 2002;168(1):67–71.

40. Beisland HO, Seland P. A prospective randomized study on neodymium-YAG laser irradiation versus TUR in the treatment of urinary bladder cancer. Scand J Urol Nephrol 1986;20(3):209–212.

41. Richie JP. Intravesical chemotherapy. Treatment selection, techniques, and results. Urol Clin North Am 1992;19(3):521–527.

42. Lamm DL. Long-term results of intravesical therapy for superficial bladder cancer. Urol Clin North Am 1992;19(3):573–580.

43. Mishina T, Oda K, Murata S, Ooe H, Mori Y. Mitomycin C bladder instillation therapy for bladder tumors. J Urol 1975;114(2):217–219.

44. Lamm DL, Torti FM. Bladder cancer, 1996. CA Cancer J Clin 1996; 46(2):93–112.

45. Flamm J. Long-term versus short-term doxorubicin hydrochloride instillation after transurethral resection of superficial bladder cancer. Eur Urol 1990;17(2):119–124.

46. Huland H, Kloppel G, Feddersen I, et al. Comparison of different schedules of cytostatic intravesical instillations in patients with superficial bladder carcinoma: final evaluation of a prospective multicenter study with 419 patients. J Urol 1990;144(1):68–71.

47. Traynelis CL, Lamm DL. Current status of intravesical therapy for bladder cancer. In: Rous SN, ed. Urology Annual. New York: Norton, 1994:113–143.

48. Pawinski A, Sylvester R, Kurth KH, et al. A combined analysis of European Organization for Research and Treatment of Cancer, and Medical Research Council randomized clinical trials for the prophylactic treatment of stage TaT1 bladder cancer. European Organization for Research and Treatment of Cancer Genitourinary Tract Cancer Cooperative Group and the Medical Research Council Working Party on Superficial Bladder Cancer. J Urol 1996; 156(6):1934–1940.

49. Morales A, Eidinger D, Bruce AW. Intracavitary Bacillus Calmette-Guerin in the treatment of super- ficial bladder tumors. 1976. J Urol 2002;167(2 pt 2):891–893.

50. Mungan NA, Witjes JA. Bacille Calmette-Guerin in superficial transitional cell carcinoma. Br J Urol 1998;82(2):213–223.

51. O'Donnell MA, Krohn J, DeWolf WC. Salvage intravesical therapy with interferon-alpha 2b plus low dose bacillus Calmette-Guerin is effective in patients with superficial bladder cancer in whom bacillus Calmette-Guerin alone previously failed. J Urol 2001;166(4): 1300–1304.

52. Debruyne FM, van der Meijden AP, Schreinemachers LM, et al. BCG-RIVM intravesical immunoprophylaxis for superficial bladder cancer. Prog Clin Biol Res 1988;269:511–524.

53. Vegt PD, Witjes JA, Witjes WP, Doesburg WH, Debruyne FM, van der Meijden AP. A randomized study of intravesical mitomycin C, bacillus Calmette-Guerin Tice and bacillus Calmette-Guerin RIVM treatment in pTa-pT1 papillary carcinoma and carcinoma in situ of the bladder. J Urol 1995;153(3 pt 2):929–933.

54. Krege S, Giani G, Meyer R, Otto T, Rubben H. A randomized multicenter trial of adjuvant therapy in superficial bladder cancer: transurethral resection only versus transurethral resection plus mitomycin C versus transurethral resection plus bacillus Calmette-Guerin. Participating Clinics. J Urol 1996;156(3):962–966.

55. Alfthan O, Jauhiainen K, Kaasinen E, Liukkonen T. Current concepts in the role of intravesical instillations in the therapy and prophylaxis of superficial transitional-cell cancer of the bladder. The Finnbladder Research Group. World J Urol 1997;15(2):89–95.

56. Lundholm C, Norlen BJ, Ekman P, et al. A randomized prospective study comparing long-term intravesical instillations of mitomycin C and bacillus Calmette-Guerin in patients with superficial bladder carcinoma. J Urol 1996;156(2 pt 1):372–376.

57. Lamm DL, Blumenstein BA, Crawford ED, et al. Randomised intergroup comparison of bacillus Calmette-Guerin immunotherapy and mitomycin C chemotherapy in superficial transitional cell carcinoma of the bladder. A Southwest Oncology Group study. Urol Oncol 1995;1:119–126.

58. Bohle A, Jocham D, Bock PR. Intravesical bacillus Calmette-Guerin versus mitomycin C for superficial bladder cancer: a formal meta-analysis of comparative studies on recurrence and toxicity. J Urol 2003;169(1):90–95.

59. Smith JA, Labsky RF, Cockett AT, Fracchia JA, Montie JE, Rowland RG. Bladder cancer clinical guidelines panel summary report on the management of nonmuscle invasive bladder cancer (stages Ta, T1 and TIS). The American Urological Association. J Urol 1999; 162(5):1697–1701.

60. Sylvester RJ, van der Meijden AP, Lamm DL. Intravesical bacillus Calmette-Guerin reduces the risk of progression in patients with superficial bladder cancer: a meta-analysis of the published results of randomized clinical trials. J Urol 2002;168(5):1964–1970.

61. Tolley DA, Parmar MK, Grigor KM, et al. The effect of intravesical mitomycin C on recurrence of newly diagnosed superficial bladder

cancer: a further report with 7 years of follow up. J Urol 1996;155(4): 1233–1238.

62. Okamura K, Ono Y, Kinukawa T, et al. Randomized study of single early instillation of (2″R)-4′-O-tetrahydropyranyl-doxorubicin for a single superficial bladder carcinoma. Cancer 2002;94(9):2363–2368.

63. Thrasher JB, Crawford ED. Complications of intravesical chemotherapy. Urol Clin North Am 1992;19(3):529–539.

64. Catalona WJ, Hudson MA, Gillen DP, Andriole GL, Ratliff TL. Risks and benefits of repeated courses of intravesical bacillus Calmette-Guerin therapy for superficial bladder cancer. J Urol 1987;137(2): 220–224.

65. Haaff EO, Dresner SM, Ratliff TL, Catalona WJ. Two courses of intravesical bacillus Calmette-Guerin for transitional cell carcinoma of the bladder. J Urol 1986;136(4):820–824.

66. Brosman SA. Experience with bacillus Calmette-Guerin in patients with superficial bladder carcinoma. J Urol 1982;128(1):27–30.

67. Gruenwald IE, Stein A, Rashcovitsky R, Shifroni G, Lurie A. A 12-versus 6-week course of bacillus Calmette-Guerin prophylaxis for the treatment of high risk superficial bladder cancer. J Urol 1997; 157(2):487–491.

68. Khanna OP, Son DL, Mazer H, et al. Multicentre study of superficial bladder cancer treated with intravesical bacillus Calmette-Guerin or Adriamycin. J Urol 1990;35(2):101–108.

69. Lamm DL, Blumenstein BA, Crissman JD, et al. Maintenance bacillus Calmette-Guerin immunotherapy for recurrent TA, T1 and carcinoma in situ transitional cell carcinoma of the bladder: a randomized Southwest Oncology Group Study. J Urol 2000;163(4): 1124–1129.

70. Martinez-Pineiro JA, Flores N, Isorna S, et al. Long-term follow-up of a randomized prospective trial comparing a standard 81 mg dose of intravesical bacille Calmette-Guerin with a reduced dose of 27 mg in superficial bladder cancer. BJU Int 2002;89(7):671–680.

71. van der Meijden AP, Sylvester RJ, Oosterlinck W, Hoeltl W, Bono AV, EORTC Genito-urinary Tract Cancer Collaborative Group. Maintenance Bacillus Calmette-Guerin for TaT1 bladder tumors is not associated with increased toxicity: results from a European Organisation for Research and Treatment of Cancer Genito-Urinary Group Phase III Trial. Eur Urol 2003;44(4):429–434.

72. Lamm DL. BCG immunotherapy for transitional-cell carcinoma in situ of the bladder. Oncology (Huntington) 1995;9(10):947–952, discussion 955.

73. Oosterlinck W, Lobel B, Jackse G, et al. EAU Recommendations 2001. Guidelines on bladder cancer. Eur Urol 2002;41(2):105–112.

74. Pham HT, Soloway MS. High-risk superficial bladder cancer: intravesical therapy for T1 G3 transitional cell carcinoma of the urinary bladder. Semin Urol Oncol 1997;15(3):147–153.

75. Birch BR, Harland SJ. The pT1 G3 bladder tumour. Br J Urol 1989; 64(2):109–116.
76. Herr HW. Progression of stage T1 bladder tumors after intravesical bacillus Calmette-Guerin. J Urol 1991;145(1):40–43.
77. Cookson MS, Sarosdy MF. Management of stage T1 superficial bladder cancer with intravesical bacillus Calmette-Guerin therapy. J Urol 1992;148(3):797–801.
78. Serretta V, Piazza S, Pavone C, Piazza B, Pavone-Macaluso M. Results of conservative treatment (transurethral resection plus adjuvant intravesical chemotherapy) in patients with primary T1, G3 transitional cell carcinoma of the bladder. Urology 1996;47(5): 647–651.
79. Stein JP, Lieskovsky G, Cote R, et al. Radical cystectomy in the treatment of invasive bladder cancer: long-term results in 1,054 patients. J Clin Oncol 2001;19(3):666–675.
80. Glashan RW. A randomized controlled study of intravesical alpha-2b-interferon in carcinoma in situ of the bladder. J Urol 1990; 144(3):658–661.
81. Boccardo F, Cannata D, Rubagotti A, et al. Prophylaxis of superficial bladder cancer with mitomycin or interferon alfa-2b: results of a multicentric Italian study. J Clin Oncol 1994;12(1):7–13.
82. Belldegrun AS, Franklin JR, O'Donnell MA, et al. Superficial bladder cancer: the role of interferon-alpha. J Urol 1998;159(6): 1793–1801.
83. Ferrari P, Castagnetti G, Pollastri CA, Ferrari G, Tavoni F, Grassi D. Chemoimmunotherapy for prophylaxis of recurrence in superficial bladder cancer: interferon-alpha 2b versus interferon-alpha 2b with epirubicin. Anticancer Drugs 1992;3(suppl 1):25–27.
84. Engelmann U, Knopf HJ, Graff J. Interferon-alpha 2b instillation prophylaxis in superficial bladder cancer—a prospective, controlled three-armed trial. Project Group Bochum-interferon and superficial bladder cancer. Anticancer Drugs 1992;suppl 1:33–37.
85. Stricker P, Pryor K, Nicholson T, et al. Bacillus Calmette-Guerin plus intravesical interferon alpha-2b in patients with superficial bladder cancer. Urology 1996;48(6):957–961.
86. Herr HW, Laudone VP, Badalament RA, et al. Bacillus Calmette-Guerin therapy alters the progression of superficial bladder cancer. J Clin Oncol 1988;6(9):1450–1455.
87. Martinez-Pineiro JA, Jimenez LJ, Martinez-Pineiro L Jr, et al. Bacillus Calmette-Guerin versus doxorubicin versus thiotepa: a randomized prospective study in 202 patients with superficial bladder cancer. J Urol 1990;143(3):502–506.
88. Lamm DL, Blumenstein BA, Crawford ED, et al. A randomized trial of intravesical doxorubicin and immunotherapy with bacille Calmette-Guerin for transitional-cell carcinoma of the bladder. N Engl J Med 1991;325(17):1205–1209.

89. Pagano F, Bassi P, Milani C, Meneghini A, Maruzzi D, Garbeglio A. A low dose bacillus Calmette-Guerin regimen in superficial bladder cancer therapy: is it effective? J Urol 1991;146(1):32–35.
90. Millan-Rodriguez F, Chechile-Toniolo G, Salvador-Bayarri J, Palou J, Vicente-Rodriguez J. Multivariate analysis of the prognostic factors of primary superficial bladder cancer. J Urol 2000;163(1):73–78.
91. Cookson MS, Herr HW, Zhang ZF, Soloway S, Sogani PC, Fair WR. The treated natural history of high risk superficial bladder cancer: 15–year outcome. J Urol 1997;158(1):62–67.
92. Pansadoro V, Emiliozzi P, de Paula F, Scarpone P, Pansadoro A, Sternberg CN. Long-term follow-up of G3T1 transitional cell carcinoma of the bladder treated with intravesical bacille Calmette-Guerin: 18–year experience. Urology 2002;59(2):227–231.
93. Patard JJ, Rodriguez A, Leray E, Rioux-Leclercq N, Guille F, Lobel B. Intravesical Bacillus Calmette-Guerin treatment improves patient survival in T1G3 bladder tumours. Eur Urol 2002;41(6):635–641.

6

Chemotherapy for Bladder Cancer

Matthew D. Galsky and Dean F. Bajorin

Key Points

1. Bladder cancer is a chemotherapy-responsive tumour.
2. MVAC was the standard, but is toxic.
3. Cisplatin and gemcitabine combination therapy is the new standard.
4. There is a role for consolidation surgery in select patients with unresectable or metastatic disease after chemotherapy.
5. Possible additive benefit to adjuvant therapy given with surgery for locally advanced disease.

Introduction

Transitional cell carcinoma (TCC) of the urinary bladder is the second most common genitourinary malignancy. Each year, over 73,000 new cases are reported in Europe and over 56,000 new cases in the United States. A substantial percentage of these patients develop metastases despite initial management for presumed localized disease, whereas others have metastases at the time of presentation. Once metastasis occurs, the median survival for patients with TCC is approximately 1 year. To improve this poor survival rate, intense efforts over the past two decades have focused on the development of active chemotherapeutic regimens for use in this disease, both in the perioperative setting and in the setting of advanced disease. Chemotherapy for advanced disease is discussed here first because of its impact on the management of early-stage disease.

Older Chemotherapeutic Regimens in Metastatic Transitional Cell Carcinoma

Older Single Agents

Cisplatin is the most active single agent in urothelial TCC. During the late 1970s, trials evaluating single-agent cisplatin were initiated in patients with advanced TCC, yielding overall response (OR) rates ranging from 26% to 65%. Although uncommon, complete response (CR) rates were also observed (5% to 16%). Subsequently, additional single agents demonstrated activity in urothelial TCC. The most active of these included methotrexate (OR 30%), doxorubicin (OR 17%), and vinblastine (OR 22%) [1,2].

Combination Chemotherapy and the Development of MVAC

Multiagent chemotherapeutic regimens were developed during the 1980s in an attempt to improve upon the results with single-agent therapy. A landmark trial reported in 1985 used the combination of methotrexate, vinblastine, Adriamycin (doxorubicin), and cisplatin (MVAC). In this trial, 24 patients with advanced or unresectable urothelial TCC were treated with MVAC [3]. Remarkably, responses were observed in 71% of those treated (95% confidence interval [CI], 53–89%), with complete clinical responses in 50% (95% CI, 30–70%). A follow-up report from the same investigators confirmed these initial results with MVAC in a larger patient population [4]. Subsequent randomized trials showed improved survival with MVAC compared to single-agent cisplatin [5] and CISCA (cisplatin, cyclophosphamide, and Adriamycin) [6].

Limitations of MVAC

Despite the superiority of MVAC in phase III trials, the limitations of this regimen were readily apparent. Although many patients responded to MVAC, median survivals were consistently reported as less than 13 months. In addition, the durability of responses with MVAC was poor, with less than 4% of patients alive and continuously disease-free at 6 years or more [7]. The most limiting factor associated with MVAC was associated toxicity. Treatment-related deaths occurred in 2% to 4% of patients. Severe toxicities such as febrile neutropenia (20% to 30%) and mucositis (10% to 20%) were also common in patients treated with this regimen. Other toxicities included decreased renal function, hearing loss, and peripheral neuropathy.

Attempts to Improve MVAC

In an attempt to decrease the toxicity and enhance the efficacy of MVAC, several investigators evaluated the use of altered doses and schedules with granulocyte colony-stimulating factor (GCSF) support. Based on the potential for enhanced survival conferred by greater drug delivery, the European Organization for Research and Treatment of Cancer (EORTC) conducted a randomized trial comparing MVAC administered every 2 weeks (with GCSF) with MVAC administered every 4 weeks [8]. Although this prospective trial showed a significantly greater CR rate (21% compared to 9%, $p = .009$) and progression-free survival (hazard ratio 0.75; 95% CI, 0.58–0.98, $p = .037$) in patients receiving the every-2-week schedule there was no significant difference in the overall survival distributions. This trial, designed to detect a 50% difference in median survival with a total of 263 patients, showed a trend toward greater survival in patients receiving more intense therapy. It is possible that a survival benefit with the dose-dense regimen may have been missed due to the small sample size. However, given the modest differences in outcome, the conventional regimen given at 4-week intervals remains the standard of care.

The Impact of Prognostic Factors

Pretreatment prognostic factors play a key role in predicting the outcome of patients with advanced TCC treated with MVAC and other cisplatin-based regimens. In a retrospective analysis, a database of 203 patients with unresectable/metastatic TCC was subjected to multivariate analysis to determine which patient characteristics predicted survival [9]. Two factors had independent prognostic significance: Karnofsky performance status (KPS) ≤80% and visceral (lung, liver, or bone) metastases. The median survival for patients with 0, 1, or 2 risk factors was 33, 13.4, and 9.3 months, respectively ($p = .0001$). Clearly, the proportion of patients in these various risk categories must be considered when compar- ing median survivals among different phase II studies. In addition, these baseline prognostic factors can be used to stratify patients in phase III trials comparing new regimens to standard therapy. Similar differences in survival have been observed in patients treated with cisplatin, gemcitabine, and paclitaxel [10].

Newer Agents/Combinations in Metastatic Transitional Cell Carcinoma

New Active Single Agents

Given the limitations with MVAC therapy, new agents had to be developed to improve long-term outcome and reduce toxicity. Recently, several agents with activity in TCC have been identified. These new agents differ from the older drugs in that they demonstrate moderate activity as both first-line and second-line therapy, more favorable toxicity profiles, and a drug metabolism that is independent of renal excretion. Of these newer agents, the most extensively studied have been gemcitabine, the taxanes, and ifosfamide.

Gemcitabine and Cisplatin: A New Standard of Care

Based on the promising activity and favorable side-effect profile of gemcitabine, trials exploring the combination of gemcitabine and cisplatin in metastatic TCC were initiated. Several phase II studies reported OR rates of 42% to 57% and CR rates of 18 to 22% [11–13]. Subsequently, a multicenter, randomized phase III trial was performed to compare gemcitabine and cisplatin (GC) with MVAC (Table 6.1) [14], in which 405 chemotherapy-naive patients were randomized to GC or standard MVAC. The CR, OR, and median survival rates were similar in both arms. Although GC was associated with more grade ≥3 anemia and thrombocytopenia, MVAC was associated with a greater incidence of neutropenic fever (14% compared to 2%), neutropenic sepsis (12% compared to 1%), grade ≥3 mucositis (22% compared to 1%), and treatment-related deaths (3% compared to 1%).

Notably, this randomized trial was not designed as an equivalence trial. However, the data can be interpreted as showing that, in terms of survival, GC is comparable to MVAC. In addition, GC appears to be associated with a more favorable risk-benefit ratio. Given the trial results and this regimen's ease of administration, GC has become widely used as a standard treatment regimen for patients with metastatic TCC.

New Cisplatin Doublets

The combinations of paclitaxel or docetaxel plus cisplatin have been explored in multiple phase II studies. In an Eastern Cooperative Oncology Group (ECOG) study, 52 patients were treated with paclitaxel $175 \, mg/m^2$ and cisplatin $75 \, mg/m^2$ every 21 days [15]. Twenty-six patients achieved an objective response (50%; 95% CI, 36–64%) with four (8%) complete responses. The toxicity of this regimen was considered moderate, with neutropenia (without fever) and neurotoxicity being most common.

Trials evaluating the combination of docetaxel and cisplatin (DC) report OR rates of 58% to 60%, with CR rates ranging from 19% to 26% [16,17]. Results of a phase III randomized trial comparing DC with MVAC plus GCSF conducted by the Hellenic Cooperative Oncology Group have recently been reported (Table 6.1) [18]. Although DC was associated with less hematologic toxicity and febrile neutropenia, response rates and survival favored the MVAC arm. The reported toxicity of the MVAC arm, administered with GCSF, was less than in previous phase III trials employing MVAC without GCSF.

Table 6.1. Randomized trials of cisplatin-based chemotherapy in advanced transitional cell carcinoma

Regimens	Reference	No. of patients	OR (%)	CR (%)	Survival (months)	p
MVAC	5	120	36	13	12.5	<.0002
Cisplatin		126	11	3	8.2	
MVAC	6	55	65	35	12.6	<.05
CISCA		55	46	25	10	
MVAC	64	86	59	24	12.5	.17
FAP		83	42	10	12.5	
MVAC	8	129	58	9	14.1	.122
HD-MVAC		134	72	21	15.5	
MVAC	14	205	46	12	14.8	.746
Gemcitabine + cisplatin		203	50	12	13.8	
MVAC	18	109	54	23	14.2	.025
Docetaxel + cisplatin		111	37	13	9.3	
*MVAC	28	44	40	13%	14.2	.41
Paclitaxel + carboplatin		41	28	3%	13.8	

MVAC, methotrexate, vinblastine, doxorubicin, cisplatin; CISCA, cyclophosphamide, cisplatin, doxorubicin; CMV, cisplatin, methotrexate, vinblastine; MV, methotrexate, vinblastine; FAP, 5-fluorouracil, interferon-alpha-2b, cisplatin; HD-MVAC, high-dose MVAC; OR, overall response; CR, complete response.
* Trial terminated early with only 85 patients, underpowered, preliminary results.

New Cisplatin Triplets

The combination of ifosfamide, paclitaxel, and cisplatin (ITP) has been studied in a phase II trial [19]. Myelosuppression was the predominant toxicity (45% grade 3 to 4 neutropenia), although the risk of febrile neutropenia was low (3.3% of all cycles). Grade 3 neuropathy and renal insufficiency occurred in 9% and 11%, respectively. Thirty of 44 assessable patients (68%; 95% CI, 52–81%) achieved a major response, with 10 complete responses (23%) and 20 partial responses (45%). The reported median survival of 20 months is among the best reported results for patients with metastatic, advanced TCC, and greater than the previously observed results with MVAC (12–13 months). This regimen has not been taken to phase III evaluation.

Other cisplatin-based triplets have been explored, the most notable of which is cisplatin, gemcitabine, and paclitaxel. In a phase I/II trial of 58 patients, this regimen resulted in 16 complete responses (28%) and 29 partial responses (50%) for an overall response proportion of 77.6% (95% CI, 60–98%) [20]. The median survival time had not been reached at the time of the report. This regimen is currently being compared with gemcitabine plus cisplatin in an international randomized phase III trial conducted by the EORTC.

New Carboplatin Doublets

Given the renal, neurologic, and auditory toxicity associated with cisplatin, it was hoped that carboplatin would prove to be equivalent to cisplatin in this disease. In a review of 327 patients with advanced, metastatic TCC treated on 13 trials with single-agent carboplatin, 14% achieved an objective response [21].

The best-studied carboplatin doublet in TCC is the combination of paclitaxel and carboplatin. Phase II trials have been performed with wide variations in the doses of paclitaxel (150 to 225 mg/m^2) and carboplatin (area under the curve [AUC] 5 to 6); not unexpectedly, the OR rates vary from 14% to 65%, and the CR rates range from 0% to 40% [22–27].

Given the promising phase II results, ECOG launched a phase III trial comparing MVAC with paclitaxel plus carboplatin; results were reported in preliminary form (Table 6.1). Because the study was terminated after $2\frac{1}{2}$ years of slow accrual [28], only 85 of the planned 330 patients were enrolled. Patients treated with MVAC had more severe myelosuppression, mucositis, and renal toxicity. Interestingly, a quality of life instrument revealed no significant differences between the two arms. At a median follow-up of 32.5 months, there was no significant difference in response rate or median survival between the two arms. However, this trial was underpowered, and definitive conclusions cannot be made due to its early termination.

The combination of gemcitabine and carboplatin has also been explored. Trials have reported OR rates ranging from 44% to 68% and CR rates ranging from 6% to 23% [29–31]. An Italian randomized phase II study comparing gemcitabine plus cisplatin versus gemcitabine plus carboplatin has been reported in preliminary form. Overall and complete response rates favored the cisplatin-containing regimen (Table 6.1) [32]. A phase III trial comparing the gemcitabine plus carboplatin regimen to the three-drug regimen of carboplatin plus methotrexate plus vinblastine has been initiated by the EORTC in patients who cannot tolerate cisplatin therapy.

New Carboplatin Triplets

Several carboplatin triplets have been studied including: paclitaxel plus carboplatin plus methotrexate [33], paclitaxel plus carboplatin plus gemcitabine [34], and methotrexate plus carboplatin plus vinblastine (M-CAV) [35]. In general, these regimens have been associated with slightly higher response proportions and slightly increased toxicity compared with historical trials of carboplatin doublets. No phase III trials have explored the activity of these triplets relative to standard therapy.

Carboplatin Compared to Cisplatin

Despite the similar response proportions of single-agent carboplatin compared to single-agent cisplatin, controversy still exists regarding the relative value of carboplatin in TCC, particularly in combination regimens. The randomized phase II trials exploring combination regimens with cisplatin compared to carboplatin consistently report higher overall and complete response rates for the cisplatin-containing regimens [32,35,36]. Consequently, in patients with advanced TCC without absolute contraindications (e.g., poor creatinine clearance, solitary kidney, poor performance status), cisplatin-based therapy should be considered the treatment of choice.

Nonplatinum Combinations

In an alternate attempt to improve the efficacy and tolerability of combination chemotherapy in advanced TCC, regimens devoid of platinum analogues have been developed. These regimens include paclitaxel plus ifosfamide [37], paclitaxel plus gemcitabine [38,39], and docetaxel plus gemcitabine [40]. Several of these trials were performed in patients who had previously received cisplatin-based therapy. Overall, these regimens were well tolerated. However, hematologic toxicity was prominent, particularly in the pretreated population. Noteworthy activity was seen with these regimens, including varying rates of complete responses, but the role of these regimens in the treatment of patients with metastatic TCC has not been defined.

Novel Therapeutic Strategies in Metastatic Transitional Cell Carcinoma

Despite the promising activity of the newer combination regimens in TCC, the majority of patients still succumb to their disease, necessitating further exploration in approaches to treatment. One novel approach is the administration of sequential dose-dense chemotherapy based on the Norton-Simon hypothesis, a mathematical prediction model of chemotherapy sensitivity derived from the Gompertzian growth rates of tumors [41]. Other studies are exploring novel targeted therapies.

Given the promising results with the Ifosfamide, pacliTaxel, and cisPlatin (ITP) regimen, a pilot study of sequenced therapy with Adriamycin (doxorubicin) and gemcitabine (AG) followed by ITP was initiated [42]. A preliminary analysis of 21 patients treated with this regimen showed a major response in 18 patients (87%; 95% CI, 71–100%) and a complete response in 43% of patients (95% CI, 22–64%) [43]. Importantly, the sequential use of ITP increased complete and partial response rates after the initial AG doublet.

Chemotherapy regimens that include new agents targeting the epidermal growth factor receptor (EGFR) pathway are also under study. The Southwest Oncology Group is evaluating trastuzumab given in combination with paclitaxel, carboplatin, and gemcitabine [44]. The selective EGFR tyrosine kinase inhibitor ZD1839, in combination with either gemcitabine/cisplatin or gemcitabine/carboplatin, is being explored as first-line therapy in two Cancer and Leukemia Group B (CALGB) trials.

Postchemotherapy Surgery in Metastatic Transitional Cell Carcinoma

The importance of postchemotherapy surgery in the setting of minimal residual disease after achieving a "near" complete response to chemotherapy has been highlighted in several analyses [45–47]. In a series of 203 patients treated on five trials with MVAC, 50 patients underwent postchemotherapy surgery for suspected or known residual disease [45]. Seventeen patients had no viable tumor found at postchemotherapy surgery. In three patients, the residual disease was unresectable. In the remaining 30, residual TCC was completely resected, resulting in a complete response to chemotherapy plus surgery. Of these 30 patients, 10 (33%) remained alive at 5 years, similar to results attained for patients achieving a complete response to chemotherapy alone. Optimal candidates for postchemotherapy resection of residual disease had prechemotherapy disease limited to the primary site or lymph nodes.

Recommendations for Treatment of Metastatic Transitional Cell Carcinoma

Over the past two decades, multiple chemotherapeutic regimens with activity in TCC have been introduced. Additionally, the importance of baseline prognostic factors, comorbidities, and postchemotherapy surgery has been recognized. Integrating this information allows the development of a rational approach to the treatment of individual patients (Fig. 6.1). Based on phase III data, GC or MVAC is recommended for patients with metastatic

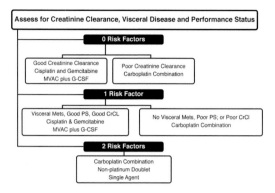

Fig. 6.1. Memorial Sloan-Kettering Cancer Center's algorithm for the management of patients with advanced/metastatic transitional cell carcinoma based on baseline prognostic factors and renal function. CrCl, creatinine clearance; Mets, metastases; PS, performance status.

TCC who can tolerate cisplatin-based therapy and who have potential for long-term benefit.

Perioperative Chemotherapy for Transitional Cell Carcinoma

Despite potentially curative surgery, approximately 50% of patients with muscle-invasive TCC develop metastases and die of disease. Given the chemosensitivity of TCC, attempts to improve survival have focused on administering chemotherapy in the perioperative setting.

Neoadjuvant Chemotherapy

Administering chemotherapy prior to surgery offers several potential advantages. Systemic therapy is initiated sooner, and patients may be able to tolerate treatment better in the pre-operative state. Furthermore, the response of the primary tumor to chemotherapy can be assessed, which is of prognostic significance. In a study of patients treated with neoadjuvant cisplatin-based therapy followed by definitive surgery, 91% of patients who responded to chemotherapy (defined as pathologic stage ≤T1) were alive at a median follow-up of 25 months compared to 37% of nonresponders [48].

Several randomized trials have explored neoadjuvant chemotherapy in TCC (Table 6.2). Although many of these trials failed to show a benefit for chemotherapy, the studies suffered from small sample size [49], suboptimal chemotherapy [50,51], premature closure [52], or inadequate follow-up time [53]. Recently, well-designed trials utilizing effective chemotherapeutic regimens have shifted the treatment paradigm in muscle-invasive disease toward the use of perioperative chemotherapy [54–56].

Intergroup trial 0080 randomized patients with T2 to T4a TCC of the bladder to radical cystectomy alone (154 patients) compared to three cycles of MVAC followed by radical cystectomy (153 patients) [55]. The use of neoadjuvant chemotherapy was associated with a higher rate of complete pathologic response (38% compared to 15%, $p < .001$). At a median follow-up of 8.7 years, improvements in median survival (77 compared to 46 months, $p = .06$) and 5-year survival (57% compared to 43%, $p = .06$) favored the neoadjuvant MVAC arm. Although approximately one third of patients treated with MVAC developed grade ≥3 hematologic or gastrointestinal toxicity, there were no treatment-related deaths, and neoadjuvant chemotherapy did not adversely impact the ability to proceed with radical cystectomy or increase adverse events related to surgery.

The Medical Research Council (MRC)/ EORTC performed a large trial in which 976 patients were enrolled and randomized to neoadjuvant cisplatin, methotrexate, and vinblastine (CMV) (491 patients) or no neoadjuvant chemotherapy (485 patients) [57]. Management of the primary tumor involved cystectomy, radiation therapy, or both. An 8% improvement in time to progression and a 5.5% difference in absolute 3-year survival (Hazard ratio (HR) = 0.85; 95% CI, 0.71–1.02) favoring the neoadjuvant chemotherapy arm were reported. The results of this trial were recently updated, and, at a median follow-up of approximately 7 years, a statistically significant improvement in survival was observed for patients who received neoadjuvant chemotherapy (HR = 0.85; 95% CI, 0.72–1.0; $p = .048$) [54]. This trial, well powered and with adequate follow-up, demonstrated both a survival benefit and improved locoregional control with neoadjuvant chemotherapy.

Table 6.2. Randomized trials of adjuvant chemotherapy

Trial organization/country	No. of patients	Treatment arms	Chemotherapy survival benefit
University of Southern California, Norris Comprehensive Cancer Center (61)	91	Cyst → CAP Cyst	Yes
University of Mainz (60)	49	Cyst → M-VAC/M-VEC Cyst	Yes
Swiss Group for Clinical Cancer Research (62)	77	Cyst → C Cyst	No
Italian Uro-Oncologic Cooperative Group (59)	83	Cyst → CM Cyst	No
Stanford University (63)	50	Cyst → CMV Cyst	No
MD Anderson Cancer Center (68)	140	MVAC → Cyst → MVAC Cyst → MVAC	*

M, methotrexate; C, cisplatin; V, vinblastine; A, (Adriamycin (doxorubicin); E, epirubicin; Cyst, cystectomy.
* In this trial, both arms received perioperative chemotherapy. Patients were randomized to receive chemotherapy both pre- and postoperatively or only postoperatively. There were no significant differences in outcome between the two arms.

A recent meta-analysis reviewed data from 2688 patients treated on 10 randomized trials evaluating neoadjuvant chemotherapy for invasive TCC [58]. Of note, this analysis did not include data from Intergroup 0080. Compared to local treatment alone, neoadjuvant platinum-based combination chemotherapy was associated with a significant benefit in overall survival (HR = 0.87; 95% CI, 0.78–0.98; p = .016), a 13% decrease in the risk of death, and a 5% absolute survival benefit at 5 years (overall survival increased from 45% to 50%). When trials utilizing single-agent cisplatin were included, the survival benefit did not achieve statistical signi- ficance (HR = 0.91; 95% CI, 0.83–1.01; p = .084).

Adjuvant Chemotherapy

As with neoadjuvant chemotherapy, administration of chemo-therapy after surgery is associated with potential advantages and disadvantages. Foremost, an adjuvant approach allows the administration of chemotherapy to be based on pathologic stage. Given the inaccuracies in clinical staging, this avoids overtreat-ment of patients who are estimated to have a reasonable out-come from surgery alone. Administration of chemotherapy after surgery also prevents delays in carrying out potentially curative surgery. The major disadvantages associated with adjuvant chemotherapy are the potential difficulties of tolerating treat-ment postoperatively and the lack of an objective means to assess response after the primary tumor is removed.

At least six randomized trials have evaluated the use of adju-vant chemotherapy following cystectomy for muscle-invasive TCC (Table 6.3) [59–63]. Although all of these trials used cis-platin-based chemotherapy and had surgery as a control arm, two trials primarily evaluated patients with bladder-confined disease [59,62]. These latter studies did not detect a survival benefit, but patients in these studies would be expected to have a better prog-nosis. Of the remaining trials, two demonstrated a survival benefit with adjuvant chemotherapy [61,62].

As a consequence of small sample size, inclusion of "good-prognosis" patients, and potentially inadequate chemotherapy, the data supporting adjuvant chemotherapy are less compelling than the data supporting neoadjuvant chemotherapy. In an effort to definitively address this issue, two large cooperative group trials are under way. The EORTC is randomizing patients with

Table 6.3. Randomized trials of neoadjuvant chemotherapy

Trial organization/country	No. of patients	Treatment arms	Chemotherapy survival benefit
MRC/EORTC (54)	975	CMV → RT/Cyst/both RT/Cyst/both	Yes
INT-0080 (55)	317	MVAC → Cyst Cyst	Yes
Nordic-1 (56)	325	C+A → RT/Cyst RT/Cyst	*Yes
Nordic-2 (65)	317	M+C → Cyst Cyst	No
Italy (GUONE) (49)	206	MVAC → Cyst Cyst	No
Italy (Genoa) (66)	104	C+5-FU → Cyst Cyst	No
Spain (CUETO) (51)	122	C → Cyst Cyst	No
Australia/UK (50)	255	C → RT RT	No
MGH/RTOG (52)	123	MCV → Cyst/RT Cyst/RT	No
GISTV (53)	171	MVEC → Cyst Cyst	No
Egypt (67)	194	Carboplatin MV → Cyst Cyst	No

MRC, Medical Research Council; EORTC, European Organization for Research and Treatment; INT, United States Intergroup; GUONE, Gruppo Uro-Oncologico del Nord Est; CUETO, Club Urologico Espagnol de Tratiemneto Oncologico; MGH, Massachussetts General Hospital; RTOG, Radiation Therapy Oncology Group; GITSV, Gruppo Italiano per lo Studio dei Tumori de la Vesicula; M, methotrexate; C, cisplatin; V, vinblastine; A, Adriamycin (doxorubicin); 5-FU, 5-fluorouracil; E, epirubicin; Cyst, cystectomy; RT, radiation therapy.
* Benefit for subset with T3–T4.

pT3-T4 or node-positive disease to immediate cisplatin-based chemotherapy (MVAC or GC) or similar chemotherapy at the time of relapse. In a trial conducted by the CALGB/Clinical Trial Support Unit (CTSU), patients meeting the same pathological criteria are randomized to either the sequential doublet of AG-TP (doxorubicin plus gemcitabine followed by paclitaxel plus cisplatin) or a conventional GC regimen.

Recommendations for Treatment of Locally Advanced Transitional Cell Carcinoma

Two large randomized trials and a meta-analysis support the concept that neoadjuvant chemotherapy for patients with muscle-invasive bladder cancer imparts a survival benefit over surgery alone. This approach should be considered for patients who are candidates for cisplatin-based combination chemotherapy and radical cystectomy. For patients who have not received neoadjuvant chemotherapy and who have extravesicular or node-positive disease following cystectomy, enrollment in a clinical trial should be encouraged. If a patient is not protocol- eligible, adjuvant cisplatin-based combination chemotherapy is a reasonable consideration.

Controversies and Outstanding Issues

1. Is cure for metastatic disease possible?
2. Is there a role for gemcitabine and cisplatin neoadjuvant therapy?
3. Do we need radiotherapy at all, or can chemotherapy be used for localised disease?

References

1. Herr H, Shipley W, Bajorin D. Cancer of the bladder. In: DeVita V Jr, Hellman S, Rosenberg S, eds. Cancer: Principles and Practice of Oncology, 6th ed. Philadelphia: Lippincott Williams & Wilkins, 2001:1396–1418.

2. Raghavan D, Shipley WU, Garnick MB, et al. Biology and management of bladder cancer. N Engl J Med 1990;322:1129–1138.

3. Sternberg CN, Yagoda A, Scher HI, et al. Preliminary results of M-VAC (methotrexate, vinblastine, doxorubicin and cisplatin) for transitional cell carcinoma of the urothelium. J Urol 1985;133: 403–407.

4. Sternberg CN, Yagoda A, Scher HI, et al. Methotrexate, vinblastine, doxorubicin, and cisplatin for advanced transitional cell carcinoma of the urothelium. Efficacy and patterns of response and relapse. Cancer 1989;64:2448–2458.

5. Loehrer PJ Sr, Einhorn LH, Elson PJ, et al. A randomized comparison of cisplatin alone or in combination with methotrexate, vinblastine, and doxorubicin in patients with metastatic urothelial carcinoma: a cooperative group study. J Clin Oncol 1992;10: 1066–1073.

6. Logothetis CJ, Dexeus F, Sella A, et al. A prospective randomized trial comparing CISCA to MVAC chemotherapy in advanced metastatic urothelial tumors. J Clin Oncol 1990;8:1050–1055.

7. Saxman SB, Propert KJ, Einhorn LH, et al. Long-term follow-up of a phase III intergroup study of cisplatin alone or in combination with methotrexate, vinblastine, and doxorubicin in patients with metastatic urothelial carcinoma: a cooperative group study. J Clin Oncol 1997;15:2564–2569.

8. Sternberg CN, de Mulder PH, Schornagel JH, et al. Randomized phase III trial of high-dose-intensity methotrexate, vinblastine, doxorubicin, and cisplatin (MVAC) chemotherapy and recombinant human granulocyte colony-stimulating factor versus classic MVAC in advanced urothelial tract tumors: European Organization for Research and Treatment of Cancer Protocol no. 30924. J Clin Oncol 2001;19:2638–2646.

9. Bajorin DF, Dodd PM, Mazumdar M, et al. Long-term survival in metastatic transitional-cell carcinoma and prognostic factors predicting outcome of therapy. J Clin Oncol 1999;17:3173–3181.

10. Bellmunt J, Albanell J, Paz-Ares L, et al. Pretreatment prognostic factors for survival in patients with advanced urothelial tumors treated in a phase I/II trial with paclitaxel, cisplatin, and gemcitabine. Cancer 2002;95:751–757.

11. von der Maase H, Andersen L, Crino L, et al. Weekly gemcitabine and cisplatin combination therapy in patients with transitional cell carcinoma of the urothelium: a phase II clinical trial. Ann Oncol 1999;10:1461–1465.

12. Kaufman D, Raghavan D, Carducci M, et al. Phase II trial of gemcitabine plus cisplatin in patients with metastatic urothelial cancer. J Clin Oncol 2000;18:1921–1927.

13. Moore MJ, Winquist EW, Murray N, et al. Gemcitabine plus cisplatin, an active regimen in advanced urothelial cancer: a phase II trial of

the National Cancer Institute of Canada Clinical Trials Group. J Clin Oncol 1999;17:2876–2881.

14. von der Maase H, Hansen SW, Roberts JT, et al. Gemcitabine and cis-platin versus methotrexate, vinblastine, doxorubicin, and cisplatin in advanced or metastatic bladder cancer: results of a large, random-ized, multinational, multicenter, phase III study. J Clin Oncol 2000;18:3068–3077.

15. Dreicer R, Manola J, Roth BJ, et al. Phase II study of cisplatin and paclitaxel in advanced carcinoma of the urothelium: an Eastern Cooperative Oncology Group Study. J Clin Oncol 2000;18:1058–1061.

16. Garcia del Muro X, Marcuello E, Guma J, et al. Phase II multicentre study of docetaxel plus cisplatin in patients with advanced urothe-lial cancer. Br J Cancer 2002;86:326–330.

17. Sengelov L, Kamby C, Lund B, et al. Docetaxel and cisplatin in metastatic urothelial cancer: a phase II study. J Clin Oncol 1998;16:3392–3397.

18. Bamias A, Aravantinos G, Deliveliotis C, et al. Docetaxel and cisplatin with granulocyte colony-stimulating factor (G-CSF) versus MVAC with G-CSF in advanced urothelial carcinoma: a multicenter, ran-domized, phase III study from the Hellenic Cooperative Oncology Group. J Clin Oncol 2004;22:1–9.

19. Bajorin DF, McCaffrey JA, Dodd PM, et al. Ifosfamide, paclitaxel, and cisplatin for patients with advanced transitional cell carcinoma of the urothelial tract: final report of a phase II trial evaluating two dosing schedules. Cancer 2000;88:1671–1678.

20. Bellmunt J, Guillem V, Paz-Ares L, et al. Phase I-II study of paclitaxel, cisplatin, and gemcitabine in advanced transitional-cell carcinoma of the urothelium. Spanish Oncology Genitourinary Group. J Clin Oncol 2000;18:3247–3255.

21. Mottet-Auselo N, Bons-Rosset F, Costa P, et al. Carboplatin and urothelial tumors. Oncology 1993;50(suppl 2):28–36.

22. Vaughn DJ, Malkowicz SB, Zoltick B, et al. Paclitaxel plus carboplatin in advanced carcinoma of the urothelium: an active and tolerable outpatient regimen. J Clin Oncol 1998;16:255–260.

23. Vaughn DJ, Manola J, Dreicer R, et al. Phase II study of paclitaxel plus carboplatin in patients with advanced carcinoma of the urothelium and renal dysfunction (E2896): a trial of the Eastern Cooperative Oncology Group. Cancer 2002;95:1022–1027.

24. Redman BG, Smith DC, Flaherty L, et al. Phase II trial of paclitaxel and carboplatin in the treatment of advanced urothelial carcinoma. J Clin Oncol 1998;16:1844–1848.

25. Pycha A, Grbovic M, Posch B, et al. Paclitaxel and carboplatin in patients with metastatic transitional cell cancer of the urinary tract. Urology 1999;53:510–515.

26. Zielinski CC, Schnack B, Grbovic M, et al. Paclitaxel and carboplatin in patients with metastatic urothelial cancer: results of a phase II trial. Br J Cancer 1998;78:370–374.

27. Small EJ, Lew D, Redman BG, et al. Southwest Oncology Group Study of paclitaxel and carboplatin for advanced transitional-cell carcinoma: the importance of survival as a clinical trial end point. J Clin Oncol 2000;18:2537–2544.

28. Dreicer R, Manola J, Roth BJ, et al. ECOG 4897: Phase III trial of methotrexate, vinblastine, doxorubicin, and cisplatin (M-VAC) versus carboplatin and paclitaxel in patients with advanced carcinoma of the urothelium [abstract]. Proc Am Soc Clin Oncol 2003;22:384(abstract 1542).

29. Carles J, Nogue M. Gemcitabine/carboplatin in advanced urothelial cancer. Semin Oncol 2001;28:19–24.

30. Bellmunt J, de Wit R, Albanell J, et al. A feasibility study of carboplatin with fixed dose of gemcitabine in "unfit" patients with advanced bladder cancer. Eur J Cancer 2001;37:2212–2215.

31. Santoro A, Santoro M, Maiorino L, et al. Phase II trial of gemcitabine plus carboplatin for urothelial transitional cell carcinoma in advanced or metastatic stage. Ann Oncol 1998;9(suppl 2):647.

32. Carteni G, Dogliotti L, Crucitta A, et al. Phase II randomised trial of gemcitabine plus cisplatin (GP) and gemcitabine plus carboplatin (GC) in patients (pts) with advanced or metastatic transitional cell carcinoma of the urothelium (TCCU) [abstract]. Proc Am Soc Clin Oncol 2003;22:384(abstract 1543).

33. Edelman MJ, Meyers FJ, Miller TR, et al. Phase I/II study of paclitaxel, carboplatin, and methotrexate in advanced transitional cell carcinoma: a well-tolerated regimen with activity independent of p53 mutation. Urology 2000;55:521–525.

34. Hussain M, Vaishampayan U, Du W, et al. Combination paclitaxel, carboplatin, and gemcitabine is an active treatment for advanced urothelial cancer. J Clin Oncol 2001;19:2527–2533.

35. Bellmunt J, Ribas A, Eres N, et al. Carboplatin-based versus cisplatin-based chemotherapy in the treatment of surgically incurable advanced bladder carcinoma. Cancer 1997;80:1966–1972.

36. Petrioli R, Frediani B, Manganelli A, et al. Comparison between a cisplatin-containing regimen and a carboplatin-containing regimen for recurrent or metastatic bladder cancer patients. A randomized phase II study. Cancer 1996;77:344–351.

37. Sweeney CJ, Williams SD, Finch DE, et al. A Phase II study of paclitaxel and ifosfamide for patients with advanced refractory carcinoma of the urothelium. Cancer 1999;86:514–518.

38. Meluch AA, Greco FA, Burris HA 3rd, et al. Paclitaxel and gemcitabine chemotherapy for advanced transitional-cell carcinoma of the urothelial tract: a phase II trial of the Minnie pearl cancer research network. J Clin Oncol 2001;19:3018–3024.

39. Sternberg CN, Calabro F, Pizzocaro G, et al. Chemotherapy with an every-2–week regimen of gemcitabine and paclitaxel in patients with transitional cell carcinoma who have received prior cisplatin-based therapy. Cancer 2001;92:2993–2998.

40. Dreicer R, Manola J, Schneider DJ, et al. Phase II trial of gemcitabine and docetaxel in patients with advanced carcinoma of the urothelium: a trial of the Eastern Cooperative Oncology Group. Cancer 2003;97:2743–2747.

41. Norton L, Simon R. The Norton-Simon hypothesis revisited. Cancer Treat Rep 1986;70:163–169.

42. Dodd PM, McCaffrey JA, Hilton S, et al. Phase I evaluation of sequential doxorubicin gemcitabine then ifosfamide paclitaxel cisplatin for patients with unresectable or metastatic transitional-cell carcinoma of the urothelial tract. J Clin Oncol 2000;18:840–846.

43. Maluf F, Hilton S, Nanus D, et al. Sequential doxorubicin/gemcitabine (AG) and ifosfamide, paclitaxel, and cisplatin (ITP) chemotherapy (AG-ITP) in patients with metastatic or locally advanced transitional cell carcinoma of the urothelium [abstract]. Proc Am Soc Clin Oncol 2000;19:342a(abstract 1344).

44. Hussain M, Smith DC, Vaishampayan U, et al. Trastuzumab (T), paclitaxel (P), carboplatin (C) and gemcitabine (G) in patients with advanced urothelial cancer and overexpression of HER-2. (NCI study #198) [abstract]. Proc Am Soc Clin Oncol 2003;22:391(abstract 1569).

45. Dodd PM, McCaffrey JA, Herr H, et al. Outcome of postchemotherapy surgery after treatment with methotrexate, vinblastine, doxorubicin, and cisplatin in patients with unresectable or metastatic transitional cell carcinoma. J Clin Oncol 1999;17:2546–2552.

46. Donat SM, Herr HW, Bajorin DF, et al. Methotrexate, vinblastine, doxorubicin and cisplatin chemotherapy and cystectomy for unresectable bladder cancer. J Urol 1996;156:368–371.

47. Miller R, Freiha F, Reese J, et al. Surgical restaging of patients with advanced transitional cell carcinoma of the urothelium treated with cisplatin, methotrexate, and vinblastine: update of the Stanford University experience [abstract]. Proc Am Soc Clin Oncol 1992;10:167.

48. Splinter TA, Scher HI, Denis L, et al. The prognostic value of the pathological response to combination chemotherapy before cystectomy in patients with invasive bladder cancer. European Organization for Research on Treatment of Cancer—Genitourinary Group. J Urol 1992;147:606–608.

49. Bassi P, Pagano F, Pappagallo G, et al. Neo- adjuvant M-VAC of invasive bladder cancer: G.U.O.N.E. multicenter phase III trial (abstract 567). Eur Urol 1998;33:142.

50. Wallace DM, Raghavan D, Kelly KA, et al. Neo-adjuvant (pre-emptive) cisplatin therapy in invasive transitional cell carcinoma of the bladder. Br J Urol 1991;67:608–615.

51. Martinez-Pineiro JA, Gonzalez Martin M, Arocena F, et al. Neoadjuvant cisplatin chemotherapy before radical cystectomy in invasive transitional cell carcinoma of the bladder: a prospective randomized phase III study. J Urol 1995;153:964–973.

52. Shipley WU, Winter KA, Kaufman DS, et al. Phase III trial of neoadjuvant chemotherapy in patients with invasive bladder cancer treated with selective bladder preservation by combined radiation therapy and chemotherapy: initial results of Radiation Therapy Oncology Group 89–03. J Clin Oncol 1998;16:3576–3583.

53. Cortesi E. Neoadjuvant treatment for locally advanced bladder cancer: a prospective randomized clinical trial [abstract]. Proc Am Soc Clin Oncol 1995;14:237(abstract 623).

54. Hall R. Updated results of a randomised controlled trial of neoadjuvant cisplatin (C), methotrexate (M) and vinblastine (V) chemotherapy for muscle-invasive bladder cancer [abstract]. Proc Am Soc Clin Oncol 2002;21:178a(abstract 710).

55. Grossman HB, Natale RB, Tangen CM, et al. Neoadjuvant chemotherapy plus cystectomy compared with cystectomy alone for locally advanced bladder cancer. N Engl J Med 2003;349:859–866.

56. Malmstrom PU, Rintala E, Wahlqvist R, et al. Five-year followup of a prospective trial of radical cystectomy and neoadjuvant chemotherapy: Nordic Cystectomy Trial I. The Nordic Cooperative Bladder Cancer Study Group. J Urol 1996;155:1903–1906.

57. Neoadjuvant cisplatin, methotrexate, and vinblastine chemotherapy for muscle-invasive bladder cancer: a randomised controlled trial. International collaboration of trialists. Lancet 1999;354:533–540.

58. Neoadjuvant chemotherapy in invasive bladder cancer: a systematic review and meta-analysis. Lancet 2003;361:1927–1934.

59. Bono AV, Benvenuti C, Reali L, et al. Adjuvant chemotherapy in advanced bladder cancer. Italian Uro-Oncologic Cooperative Group. Prog Clin Biol Res 1989;303:533–540.

60. Stockle M, Meyenburg W, Wellek S, et al. Advanced bladder cancer (stages pT3b, pT4a, pN1 and pN2): improved survival after radical cystectomy and 3 adjuvant cycles of chemotherapy. Results of a controlled prospective study. J Urol 1992;148:302–306.

61. Skinner DG, Daniels JR, Russell CA, et al. The role of adjuvant chemotherapy following cystectomy for invasive bladder cancer: a prospective comparative trial. J Urol 1991;145:459–464.

62. Studer UE, Bacchi M, Biedermann C, et al. Adjuvant cisplatin chemotherapy following cystectomy for bladder cancer: results of a prospective randomized trial. J Urol 1994;152:81–84.

63. Freiha F, Reese J, Torti FM. A randomized trial of radical cystectomy versus radical cystectomy plus cisplatin, vinblastine and methotrexate chemotherapy for muscle invasive bladder cancer. J Urol 1996; 155:495–499.

64. Siefker-Radtke AO, Millikan RE, Tu SM, et al. Phase III trial of fluorouracil, interferon alpha-2b, and cisplatin versus methotrexate, vinblastine, doxorubicin, and cisplatin in metastatic or unresectable urothelial cancer. J Clin Oncol 2002;20:1361–1367.

65. Malmstrom PU, Rintala E, Wahlqvist R, et al. Neoadjuvant cisplatin-methotrexate chemotherapy of invasive bladder cancer: Nordic cystectomy trial 2: XIVth Congress of the European Association of Urology [abstract]. Eur Urol 1999;35(suppl 2):60(abstract 238).

66. Curotto A, Martorana G, Venturini M, et al. Multicenter randomized study on the comparison between radical cystectomy alone and neoadjuvant alternate chemoradiotherapy before radical cystectomy: Assessment over 104 patients. In: Gluliani L, Puppo P, eds. Urology. Genova: Monduzzi, 1992:489–493.

67. Abol-Enein H, El-Mekresh M, El-Baz M, et al. Neoadjuvant chemotherapy in treatment of invasive transitional bladder cancer: a controlled prospective randomized study [abstract]. Br J Urol 1997;80(suppl 2):49(abstract 191).

68. Millikan R, Dinney C, Swanson D, et al. Integrated therapy for locally advanced bladder cancer: final report of a randomized trial of cystectomy plus adjuvant M-VAC versus cystectomy with both preoperative and postoperative M-VAC. J Clin Oncol 2001;19:4005–4013.

7

Cytokine and Angiogenesis Inhibitors

Simon Chowdhury, Martin Gore, and
Timothy G. Eisen

Key Points

1. Cytokines are modestly effective.
2. Prognostic factors delineate response rates to cytokines.
3. There is a survival advantage to nephrectomy in patients with metastastic disease who go on to receive immunotherapy.
4. The response to interferon is usually transient.
5. Complete responses to interleukin-2 are rare but may be durable.
6. Kinase inhibitors have significant benefits.

Introduction

Renal cell carcinoma is an important malignancy accounting for approximately 3% of all adult cancers [1]. The incidence of renal cell carcinoma has been steadily and significantly increasing over the past two decades, with worldwide mortality expected to exceed 100,000 [2]. A significant proportion of patients with localized disease can be cured by nephrectomy; however, at presentation approximately 50% of patients have locally advanced or metastatic disease [3]. The outlook for these patients remains poor, with a 5-year survival of less than 10% [2].

Renal cell carcinoma is an inherently chemoresistant tumor. There have been many trials of single agent and combination chemotherapy regimens; however, response rates are low and characteristically of short duration. Yagoda and colleagues [4], in a review of 4093 adequately treated patients in 83 phase II chemotherapy trials published between 1983 and 1993, showed an overall response rate of only 6%. Thus, there is no role for chemotherapy alone in the treatment of renal cell carcinoma, but there have been improvements in survival as a result of the development of cytokine therapy.

Prognostic Factors

Metastatic renal cell carcinoma encompasses a heterogeneous group of patients, and it is important to identify prognostic factors that predict survival. Assessment of these factors can assist in decisions regarding patient management as well as categorizing patients in clinical studies, thus aiding trial interpretation. The initial analysis of these factors was carried out by Elson and colleagues [5]. This retrospective study looked at 610 patients treated in the Eastern Cooperative Group (ECOG) phase II trials for advanced renal cell carcinoma between 1975 and 1984. They identified the following risk factors (see below), which enabled them to stratify patients into appropriate risk groups (Table 7.1):

1. ECOG performance status (performance status 1, 2, and 3 counting as one, two, and three risk factors respectively)
2. Recent diagnosis (<1 year)
3. More than one metastatic site
4. Recent weight loss
5. Prior cytotoxic chemotherapy

Other studies analyzing prognostic factors in patients with metastatic renal cell carcinoma have defined different parameters, but consistently performance status and a measure of disease extent appear to be important indicators of survival [6–8].

A retrospective study by Motzer and colleagues [9] looked at the relationship between pretreatment clinical features and survival in 670 patients with advanced renal cell carcinoma treated in Memorial Sloan-Kettering Cancer Center clinical trials

Table 7.1. Prognostic groups and their impact on survival

Risk group	No. of risk factors	No. of patients	Median survival (months)
1	0–1	113	12.8
2	2	141	7.7
3	3	151	5.3
4	4	123	3.4
5	5	82	2.1

From Elson et al. [5].

between 1975 and 1996. The following five pretreatment features were associated with a shorter survival in the multivariate analysis:

1. Low Karnofsky performance status (<80%)
2. High serum lactate dehydrogenase ($\geq$1.5 times upper limit of normal)
3. Low hemoglobin (less than the lower limit of normal)
4. High corrected serum calcium ($\geq$10 mg/dL)
5. Absence of prior nephrectomy

Using these factors the authors stratified patients into three separate risk groups (Table 7.2). A recent study from the same group has analyzed prognostic factors in previously treated patients with metastatic renal cell carcinoma [10]. More patients are entering second-line trials of therapy, and thus stratification of these patients is becoming increasingly important. A total of 251 patients treated in 29 consecutive trials between 1975 and 2002 were analyzed. Median survival for the 251 patients was 10.2 months and differed according to the year of treatment, with patients treated after 1990 showing longer survival. The median overall survival for this group was 12.7 months. The purpose of this study was to establish prognostic factors for this group of patients, who had all received prior cytokine therapy (interferon and/or interleukin-2), and thus establish prognostic factors for current clinical trial design. Pretreatment features associated with a poorer prognosis in the multivariate analysis were low Karnofsky performance status (<80%), low hemoglobin (less than the lower limit of normal), and high corrected serum

Table 7.2. Prognostic groups and their impact on survival

Risk group	Risk factors	Percent of patients	Median survival (months)
Favorable	0	25	20
Intermediate	1–2	53	10
Poor	3 or more	22	4

From Motzer et al. [9].

calcium ($\geq$10 mg/dL). Although these and the previously mentioned prognostic factors are useful in aiding management decisions and subsequently in interpreting trial results, they are not prescriptive, and each patient should be assessed individually.

It is also important to be aware that histologically renal cell carcinoma is a diverse group of tumors, including clear cell, papillary, chromophobe, collecting duct and unclassified cell types. Of these, clear cell is the most common subtype, accounting for approximately 70% of cases. The importance of distinguishing between these different histologies is shown by the fact that metastatic non–clear cell carcinoma is characterized by an increased resistance to systemic therapy and poorer survival [11].

Immunotherapy

The immune system has evolved to detect and destroy molecules or pathogens that are recognized as "non-self" but not to react to host tissues. Manipulation of the immune system for cancer treatment attempts either to make the tumor appear more foreign when compared to normal tissues or to magnify host immune responses to tumors. The variable natural history of metastatic renal cell carcinoma, and occasional observed spontaneous regression suggest a role for the immune system in control of tumor progression and provide a rationale for the use of immunotherapy. To improve on the current rate of success seen with immunotherapy, some important issues need to be addressed:

- Why are certain cancers more susceptible?
- Are there factors that predict responsiveness?
- What mechanisms underlie resistance and development of resistance?

Studies addressing some of these points are already underway and have already demonstrated T cell [12,13] and dendritic cell dysfunction [14] in this patient group.

Further evidence of an innate antitumor response is provided by the fact that tumor-infiltrating lymphocytes can be detected in renal cell carcinoma tissue [15]. In addition, the presence of cytotoxic T lymphocytes (CTLs) within this population suggests the presence of antigens for their development, and analysis of CTLs has revealed four separate antigens defined in renal cell carcinoma [16]. The ways in which these discoveries can be harnessed to improve current therapies are under investigation.

Cytokine Therapy

Cytokines are soluble proteins produced by mononuclear cells of the immune system that act as messengers between cells. They have a wide range of biological effects, particularly on cells of the immune system and hemopoietic lineage. The cytokine network is complicated, and this complexity makes it difficult to know how intervention with one cytokine will affect the production of others. Cytokines may act antagonistically, and thus an intervention planned to enhance a particular branch of the immune response could actually lead to suppression. Another difficulty is in providing adequate dose levels and maintaining them over a clinically significant period.

Despite these difficulties, cytokine therapy has become an integral part of biological therapy for metastatic renal cell carcinoma. Their activity is shown in separate survival analyzes by Fossa et al. [8] (Table 7.3), Jones et al. [7] (Table 7.4), and Motzer et al. [9]. In the analysis by Motzer et al., cytokine therapy (interferon-α [IFN-α] and/or interleukin-2 [IL-2]) was shown to have a statistically significant survival advantage: 12.9 months versus 6.3 months for chemotherapy; $p < .0001$). The benefit of cytokine therapy appeared to be greatest in those with more favorable

Table 7.3. The impact of interferon-alpha on survival in renal cancer

Prognostic group	Median survival ECOG (months)	Median survival IFN-α (months)	p value
Good	11.4	23.3	<.001
Moderate	8.1	11.3	.1014
Poor	5.0	6.9	NS

ECOG, Eastern Cooperative Oncology Group; NS, nonsignificant.
From Fossa et al. [8].

Table 7.4. The impact of interleukin-2 (IL-2) on survival in renal cancer

Prognostic group	Median survival ECOG (months)	Median survival IL-2 (months)	p value
Good	12.6	20.4	.0001
Moderate	7.2	11.4	.0013
Poor	5.6	6.3	NS

From Jones et al. [7].

prognostic disease. The median survival times for favorable-risk, intermediate-risk and poor-risk patients were 27, 12, and 6 months for those treated with cytokines and 15, 7, and 3 months for those treated with chemotherapy, respectively [17].

Negrier and colleagues [18] have identified factors predictive of rapid progression of patients with metastatic renal cell carcinoma treated by cytokines. They looked at the records of 782 patients enrolled in trials using cytokine regimens by the Groupe Francais d'Immunotherapie. Four independent factors predictive of rapid progression under cytokine treatment were identified: hepatic metastases, short interval from primary to metastases (<1 year), more than one metastatic site, and elevated neutrophil counts. Patients who had at least three of these factors have ⩾80% probability of rapid progression despite treatment, and this may well influence treatment choices.

The Role of Nephrectomy Before Cytokine Therapy

The role of nephrectomy in metastatic renal cell carcinoma remains controversial. Distant metastases may regress after nephrectomy. However, because the rate of regression is low (<1%) [19], the theory that nephrectomy causes regression is unproven, and morbidity is associated with nephrectomy, it is not indicated for this purpose. Historically there was a role for nephrectomy under the following circumstances:

1. Large symptomatic primary tumor associated with small to moderate volume metastatic disease. Local symptoms such as pain and hemorrhage are well palliated by nephrectomy. Nephrectomy has a lower morbidity than radiotherapy or embolization and may also improve or completely reverse systemic constitutional symptoms by substantially reducing the tumor burden.

2. Large asymptomatic primary tumor associated with small metastatic disease, where it is likely that the patient will develop local symptoms before symptoms related to metastases occur. We have called this "prophylactic palliation."

3. Patients with a solitary metastasis, where prolonged survival can occur following a combination of nephrectomy and resection of the metastasis [20].

These clinical scenarios in our view are still valid reasons to perform a nephrectomy in the presence of metastatic disease. However, recently randomized trials have provided us with data that argues more strongly for nephrectomy prior to cytokine therapy in the setting of metastatic disease. Certain immunotherapy trials have required patients to have a nephrectomy prior to trial entry. The rationale for this approach is that reduction of tumor burden may increase the likelihood of response. This biological argument is supported by animal data showing that the large bulk of primary tumor is either immunosuppressive or acts as an "immunological sink" with suppression of cell-mediated immunity that is reversed upon removal of the primary tumor [21,22]. Improvements in human immune responses have also been demonstrated postnephrectomy [23]. Removal of the primary also gives the possibility of harvesting tumor infiltrating lymphocytes and tumor cells for use in experimental therapies.

The role of cytoreductive surgery in relation to cytokine therapy for metastatic renal cell carcinoma has been addressed by three studies. In the first of these studies Pantuck and colleagues [24] conducted a retrospective analysis of patients with renal cell carcinoma treated with nephrectomy at UCLA. Patients with metastatic disease treated with nephrectomy prior to IL-2 therapy had significantly improved survival compared to patients treated with IL-2 alone (IL-2 alone; 1- and 2-year survival 29% and 4%, nephrectomy followed by IL-2 67% and 44%, respectively). Like any retrospective analysis there is a concern about selection bias, and patients who are not offered nephrectomy are often those with worse prognostic factors.

However, these results have been supported by two randomized phase III trials. In the larger of these studies, the Southwest Oncology Group (SWOG) trial 8949 assessed whether nephrectomy prior to treatment with IFN-α prolonged survival. A total of 246 patients with metastatic renal cell carcinoma were randomized to radical nephrectomy followed by IFN-α or to IFN-α alone. This trial showed that nephrectomy prior to systemic IFN-α gave a significant survival benefit (median survival: IFN-α alone: 8.1 months; nephrectomy followed by IFN-α 11.1 months, $p = .05$) [25].

A similar positive result was obtained in a simultaneous phase III trial conducted by the European Organization for Research and Treatment of Cancer (EORTC) that randomized 85 patients into the same treatment arms as SWOG 8949 [26]. Again nephrectomy preceding treatment with IFN-α significantly improved survival (median survival: IFN-α alone: 7 months; nephrectomy followed by IFN-α 17 months, hazard ratio 0.54, 95% confidence interval [CI] 0.31–0.94). This confirmatory result, even in a smaller study, strengthens the results from the SWOG trial and increases the likelihood that the differences seen in survival are due to nephrectomy.

The combined updated analysis of these two trials has just been published, and yielded a median survival of 13.6 months for nephrectomy followed by IFN-α versus 7.8 months for IFN-α alone [27]. This represents a 31% reduction in the risk of death ($p = .002$). Thus, cytoreductive nephrectomy appears to significantly improve overall survival in patients with metastatic renal cell carcinoma treated with IFN-α. This effect was independent of performance status, the site of metastases, and the presence of measurable disease. Although the result is statistically significant, the overall survival advantage is only 5.8 months, and as the authors state, emphasizes the need for more potent immunotherapy in the setting of cytoreductive nephrectomy.

It is important to stress that in both trials patients were highly selected initially by high performance status (0 or 1). The EORTC also excluded patients whose responses they felt would not be improved by removal of the primary tumor. This included disease distribution (bone, liver, contralateral kidney), extent of metastases, non–clear cell histology, and patients at risk of rapid worsening of symptoms after surgery. Although the Flanigan et al. [27] study does not comment on such additional exclusion factors, it would appear likely that further selection occurred, as it took 7 years to accrue 246 patients from 80 institutions at an average of one patient recruited every 2 years from each institution. Authors from both studies recommend nephrectomy before immunotherapy as a standard treatment for patients with metastatic renal cell carcinoma. Although we would concur with this conclusion, it is important to stress that these results are not applicable to the overall population of patients with metastatic renal cell carcinoma especially those of lower performance statuses and other negative prognostic features.

A concern especially when considering postnephrectomy systemic therapies is the morbidity associated with surgery. Improved surgical techniques mean that a high proportion of patients will proceed to systemic therapies postoperatively. For example, in the EORTC study only one patient randomized to surgery failed to receive postoperative IFN-α. A report from Naitoh and colleagues [28] suggests that even patients with locally advanced disease (T3 with vena caval thrombi) can safely undergo nephrectomy, with 80% subsequently receiving immunotherapy. Improvements in operative technique are likely to further decrease operative morbidity and improve the number of patients eligible for systemic therapies as well as the time to commencement of such therapies.

Interferons

Interferons were the first cytokines to be identified as a family of proteins produced by cells in response to viral infection or stimulation with double-stranded RNA, antigens, or mitogens [29].

They have a wide range of actions including immunomodulatory activity, antiviral activity, antiproliferative effects on normal and malignant cells, inhibition of angiogenesis, and enhancement of expression of a variety of cell surface antigens. Their direct antiproliferative activity is thought to play a major part in their antitumor effects, but other actions may prove important. No definitive mechanism has been identified to explain how interferons inhibit the growth of tumors, except that they prolong the G0/G1 phase of the cell cycle. This heterogeneous group of glycoproteins are classified into α, β, and γ types.

The majority of clinical research has centered on IFN-α, as it appears to have the greatest activity. Most studies have reported response rates of 15% to 20% with IFN-α and median response durations of 6 to 10 months [29]. A dosing range of 5 to 10 million IU/m^2 given intramuscularly or subcutaneously has been most commonly used, although an optimum treatment regimen or duration has not been defined. An alternative form is pegylated interferon (PEG-IFN) where IFN-α is modified by the addition of a branched polyethylene-glycol (PEG) molecule. This results in sustained absorption and prolonged half-life after subcutaneous administration, allowing weekly administration, although it may cause longer duration side effects. Two recent multicenter phase II trials have reported comparable results. Motzer and colleagues [30] reported a response rate of 13% (five of 40 previously untreated patients; one complete response [CR], and four partial responses [PRs]) [30]. Bukowski and colleagues [31] reported a response rate of 14% in 44 previously untreated patients.

Despite numerous clinical trials, it was not known until recently whether therapy with IFN-α improved survival. A Medical Research Council (MRC) study addressed this issue by comparing subcutaneous IFN-α (10 mU subcutaneously [sc] three times per week for 12 weeks; $n = 174$) with oral medroxyprogesterone acetate (MPA) (300 mg daily for 12 weeks; $n = 176$) [32]. The trial was stopped in November 1997 when data were available for 335 patients. There was a 28% reduction in the risk of death in the IFN-α group (hazard ratio 0.72; 95% CI, 0.55–0.94; $p = .017$). Interferon-α gave an improvement in 1-year survival of 12% (MPA 31%, IFN-α 43%) and an improvement in median survival of 2.5 months (MPA 6 moths, IFN-α 8.5 months). A reanalysis of the mature data confirms the survival advantage in patients treated with IFN-α (2-year survival improvement 9%;

13% MPA and 22% with IFN-α) [33]. As the authors suggest, the small benefit of IFN-α should be weighed against potential toxicity. However, IFN-α should become the standard control arm in future trials for advanced renal cell carcinoma.

Support for this view comes from the Cochrane Review of immunotherapy for advanced renal cell carcinoma [34]. The results from six studies (involving 963 patients) showed that IFN-α is superior to controls (odds ratio for death at 1 year = 0.67; 95% CI, 0.5–0.89). The weighted average median improvement in survival was 2.6 months. The reviewers concluded that IFN-α provides a survival benefit when compared to other commonly used treatments, and that it should be considered as the control arm in future studies of systemic agents.

Unlike chemotherapy, the time taken to respond to interferons may be prolonged and varies widely. Most patients who are going to respond will have done so by 3 to 4 months, and it is unusual for patients who progress on interferons to subsequently respond. However, there are reports of responses only starting to occur at 6 and 9 months. There is also the question of treatment duration in patients with either stabilization of disease or a partial or complete remission. Our current practice is to continue treatment indefinitely for those patients with stable disease or in remission, provided they are able to tolerate the side effects and treatment is stopped as soon as progressive disease occurs. Toxicity associated with interferon therapy includes flu-like symptoms, rashes, gastrointestinal complaints, liver dysfunction, neurological complaints, and fatigue, and are highly dose and schedule dependent. It is possible to alleviate some symptoms by administration at night and by the use of paracetamol and/or nonsteroidal antiinflammatory drugs prior to administration.

The benefit observed with IFN-α appears to be greatest in patients with good or moderate prognostic disease [17]. Table 7. 3 shows the impact of IFN-α on survival in renal cancer; it is derived from a case-control study involving 231 patients. Controls were obtained from an ECOG database of patients treated in non-biological therapy trials.

Attempts have been made to augment the activity of IFN-α with 13-cis-retinoic acid (13-CRA). The rationale for this approach was the observation that 13-CRA increased the antiproliferative effects of IFN-α in several interferon-sensitive renal carcinoma cell lines [35]. An initial phase II trial showed a promising response rate of 30% [36], and so a randomized phase III study was conducted to see whether the addition of 13-CRA to IFN-α was superior to IFN-α alone [37]. Response proportion and survival did not increase with the combination, and so this cannot be recommended in the treatment of metastatic renal cell carcinoma.

A trial of IFN-γ versus placebo in metastatic renal cell carcinoma showed similar response rates in both groups (4.4% interferon versus 6.6% placebo; $p = .54$) [38]. The median time to progression was 1.9 months in both arms of the study ($p = .49$), and there was no significant difference in median survival (12.2 months with interferon versus 15.7 months with placebo; $p = .52$). The addition IFN-γ to IFN-α has also been tested in a randomized phase III trial [39]. An interim analysis showed a response rate of 13% (7/53; two CR and five PR) in the IFN-α monotherapy arm and 4% (2/45; one CR and one PR) in the combination arm ($p = .17$). These results show that not all cytokines have activity in metastatic renal cell carcinoma and demonstrate the need for randomized trials.

Interleukin-2

Interleukin-2 (IL-2) is the other cytokine that has shown significant activity against renal cell carcinoma. IL-2 is produced primarily by T cells; it has no intrinsic antitumor activity, but it has a wide range of actions and plays a central role in immune regulation. Its primary action is to stimulate growth of activated T cells that bear the IL-2 receptor; it also potentiates the activity of cytotoxic T cells and production of other cytokines.

The initial work on IL-2 was carried out by Rosenberg's group at the National Cancer Institute using a high-dose intravenous (IV) bolus of IL-2. They reported on 255 patients with renal cell carcinoma treated in seven separate phase II trials using high-dose bolus single-agent IL-2 [40]. An update from this group shows an overall response rate of 15% (7% CR and 8% PR) [41]. Responses were noted in all sites of disease including bone, intact primary tumors, and visceral metastases, and in patients with large tumor burdens. The major response duration for all complete responses has yet to be reached, but is at least 80 months (range 7 to 131 months). Median duration of response for partial responders is 20 months. Median survival for all 255 patients is

16.3 months, with 10% to 20% of patients estimated to be alive 5 to 10 years after treatment.

A major limitation in the use of high-dose bolus IL-2 is its significant toxicity. The toxicity manifests itself as a vascular leak syndrome with fluid retention, edema, and ultimately multiorgan dysfunction. The most common major toxicities seen are hypotension and oliguria, which often require vasopressor support (in the previous reported series ⩾50% of the 255 patients required vasopressors). This toxicity limits the number of patients who are suitable for treatment and limits the use of IL-2 to centers able to provide appropriate supportive measures. Other important toxicities affect the cardiovascular, neurological, hematological, and gastrointestinal systems.

The high-dose IV bolus IL-2 regimen has been compared with a lower dose IV bolus (regimen: 1/10th dose) to see if toxicity could be reduced while maintaining efficacy [42]. A total of 125 patients with metastatic renal cell carcinoma were randomized; interestingly the received dose intensity difference was less than 10 because patients were able to tolerate more doses in the lower dose arm. Response rates between the two arms were comparable: 15% in the lower dose arm (7% CR and 8% PR) and 20% in the high-dose arm (3% CR and 17% PR). Toxicity as expected was considerably reduced in the lower dose arm. Thus it appears that low-dose IV bolus IL-2 is an acceptable alternative to the standard high-dose IV bolus IL-2; however, at present the response duration and survival data remain preliminary, and further patients are being accrued to this study.

The definitive results of this trial have recently been published with the full accrual of 400 patients, all with active therapy completed and a median follow-up of 7.4 years [43]. After randomly assigning 117 patients, the trial was expanded to include a third arm of low-dose subcutaneous IL-2, and an additional 283 patients were recruited. Separate analyzes were performed for the two-arm comparison of patients randomly assigned to receive high-versus low-dose IV IL-2 and the three-arm comparison that included the low-dose subcutaneous arm.

Toxicity was markedly reduced when low-dose (either regimen) rather than high-dose IL-2 was given, particularly with respect to hypotension, disorientation or confusion, and thrombocytopenia. In the two-arm comparison of high-dose versus low-dose IV IL-2, there were 11 complete responses (7%) and 22 partial responses (14%) to high-dose therapy, and for low-dose therapy there were six complete responses (4%) and 13 partial responses (9%; for overall response rate $p = .048$). For the three-arm comparison, the response rates for high-dose IV, low-dose IV, and low-dose subcutaneous IL-2 were 21% (six CR and 14 PR), 11% (one CR and nine PR), and 10% (two CR and seven PR), respectively. The difference in response rates between high-dose IV and low-dose subcutaneous was significant ($p = .033$). Response durations indicated a trend toward more complete and durable responses with high-dose IV IL-2. Eight of the 11 patients who had complete tumor regression with high-dose IL-2 remain in ongoing complete response at a median follow-up of 9.3 years.

There were no significant differences in overall survival at a median follow-up of 7.4 years for all patients and with 21% patients still alive. However, the survival of patients completely responding to high- and low-dose IV IL-2 differs significantly ($p = .04$). Although the small numbers of patients who achieve a complete response makes interpretation of these data difficult. As the authors state, the value of IL-2 in the treatment of metastatic renal cell cancer lies in the fact that for small numbers of patients it can be curative. Thus, regimens that aim to limit toxicity should not comprise its activity. In the absence of significant differences in survival, low-dose IL-2 (either IV or subcutaneously) remains a viable therapeutic option, especially for patients with significant comorbidities. This study again highlights the need to define pretreatment features that identify patients likely to respond to therapy. The improvement in survival seen in patients who achieve complete responses to high- as opposed to low-dose IV IL-2 raises the question of the benefit of dose intensification either de novo or in patients responding to low-dose IL-2.

In addition, IL-2 can also be injected subcutaneously, which allows prolonged outpatient therapy to be given. A summary of phase II trials of single-agent subcutaneous IL-2 shows a response rate of 17.9% in 190 patients (3.2% CR, 14.7% PR) [44]. Although the response rate appears comparable to intravenous administration, the database is small, and the durability of responses and hence the effect on survival are yet to be established.

Interleukin-2 can also be administered by continuous venous infusion (CVI). This method of delivery takes into account the short half-life of IL-2 (12.9 minutes). Overall response rates vary considerably, but in an overview of published trials using CVI IL-

2, a response rate of 13.6% is seen in 789 patients (2.7% CR, 10.9% PR) [44]. Complete responses are thus seen and median response duration is similar to high-dose bolus infusions. Toxicity using CVI IL-2 appears lower than that seen with the high-dose bolus strategy.

The optimal dose, schedule, and route of administration for IL-2 in patients with renal cell carcinoma have yet to be defined. Response rates appear similar with all three methods of administration, although data on response duration and overall survival are awaited before definitive comparisons can be made.

Lindsey and colleagues [45] have investigated the impact of the number of treatment courses of high-dose bolus IL-2 in patients with metastatic renal cell carcinoma. Of the 201 patients treated there was a response rate of 19% (18 CR and 20 PR). Among responders 34 out of 38 achieved at least a PR after their first course of IL-2; 37 of these 38 responders to IL-2 had achieved at least a PR after two courses of therapy. The one exception was a patient who had achieved a minor response after two courses and was re-treated and achieved a CR. Based on this analysis, the authors recommend that patients with an objective response to treatment with high-dose bolus IL-2 receive additional treatment courses until either CR or IL-2 tolerance develops. Patients with no objective response after two cycles should have no further treatment.

The impact of single-agent IL-2 on survival has not been demonstrated in a randomized phase III trial. However, Jones and colleagues [7] compared the survival of 327 patients receiving CVI IL-2 to a set of matched controls from the ECOG database. Treatment with IL-2 was associated with a prolongation of survival in patients with good or moderate prognostic disease (Table 7.4).

Initial experience with high-dose IL-2 in renal cell carcinoma involved its administration with lymphocyte-activated killer (LAK) cells. Overall results with IL-2 and LAK cells are similar to those seen with IL-2 alone [46]. In a prospective randomized trial of high-dose IV bolus IL-2 alone or with LAK cells conducted by Rosenberg and colleagues [46], no significant difference in overall survival was seen between the two groups, and this approach is no longer used.

Another strategy used to potentially enhance the activity of IL-2 is to give it in combination with tumor infiltrating lymphocytes (TILs), which are found in high numbers in renal cell carcinoma and can be expanded ex vivo in the presence of IL-2. Murine and clinical models have suggested synergy between TILs and IL-2 to activate the cellular immune response and cause tumor regression. In a pilot study by Figlin and colleagues [47] involving 55 patients treated with nephrectomy followed by TILs plus low-dose IL-2, 19/55 patients (34.5%) responded and 5 (9%) achieved a complete response. In the subgroup of 23 patients, who received CD8$^+$ TILs, the overall response rate was 43.5%. In view of this encouraging single-institution study, a randomized multicenter study was conducted to compare CD8$^+$ TILs plus low-dose IL-2 versus low-dose IL-2 alone [48]. All patients underwent nephrectomy from which tissue was obtained to generate CD8$^+$ TILs. In the intention-to-treat analysis, there was no significant difference in response rate (9.4% vs. 11.4%) and 1-year survival rate (55% vs. 47%) in the TIL/IL-2 and IL-2 groups, respectively. However, it is difficult to draw meaningful conclusions from this study, as only 48% of patients who were randomized to the TIL/IL-2 arm actually received TIL therapy. The major cause for this was cell-processing failures with insufficient yield of viable cells, although in the pilot study 96% of intended patients were treated with CD8$^+$ TILs (23 of 24).

In patients who have initially responded to IL-2, there remains the possibility to re-treat with IL-2 at relapse. In a study from Rosenberg's group [49], 48 patients with either metastatic renal cell carcinoma or melanoma who had initially achieved a partial or complete response to IL-2–based immunotherapy were re-treated at relapse. Only two of the 48 patients responded, and so it seems that re-treatment rarely produces a second response, and alternative approaches should be considered in these patients.

Interleukin-2 and Interferon-α

Synergistic antitumor effects of combining IL-2 and IFN-α are seen in murine tumor models and provide a rationale for their use in the clinical setting. The exact mechanisms of synergy are unknown, but it is possible that administration of IFN-α may increase the immunogenicity of tumor cells via an enhancement of their histocompatibility and tumor-associated antigens, thus increasing their lysis by CTLs, the number of which are increased by IL-2.

Clinical trials investigating IFN-α and IL-2 combination therapy have used different routes of administration, treatment schedules, cytokine doses, patient selection and response criteria. Thus comparisons are difficult; however, an overview of phase I and II trials showed a response rate of 20% in over 1400 patients with metastatic renal cell carcinoma [44], with approximately 25% of responders achieving a complete response.

A French multicenter randomized trial investigated the efficacy of single-agent versus combination IL-2 and IFN-α [50]. A total of 425 patients were randomized to receive either IL-2 alone (18 mU/m^2/day CVI on days 1 to 5 and days 12 to 15, as two induction cycles followed by four maintenance cycles), IFN-α alone (18 mU sc 3 times/week for 10 weeks), or a combination of IL-2 and IFN-α (same dose IL-2, but only 6 mU IFN-α three times/week, during the two induction and subsequent maintenance periods). Intention-to-treat analysis showed a significantly improved response rate after 10 weeks (IL-2: 6.5%; IFN-α: 7.5%; IL-2 and IFN-α: 20%; $p < .01$) and 1-year event-free survival (IL-2: 15%; IFN-α: 12%; IL-2 and IFN-α: 20%; $p = .01$) for patients receiving combination therapy. However, there was no significant difference in overall survival between the three groups (IL-2: 12 months; IFN-α: 13 months; IL-2 and IFN-α: 17 months; $p = .55$). Importantly, as with the case-control studies of IFN-α and IL-2, this study identified a subgroup of patients who had little chance of benefiting from treatment. These patients had more than one metastatic site, liver involvement, an interval between diagnosis of the primary tumor and development of metastases of less than 1 year, or a performance status of ≥ 1.

This study also assessed the benefit of crossover therapy after failure of IL-2 or IFN-α [51]. A total of 113 patients with progressive disease after first-line treatment received either IFN-α ($n = 48$) or IL-2 ($n = 65$) as second-line treatment. Only four patients achieved a PR (one with IFN-α; three with IL-2); of these patients, three had stable disease or had responded to first-line treatment. All partial responders had a performance status of 0 and pulmonary metastases. Only one patient with confirmed disease progression after IL-2 subsequently responded to IFN-α. Thus in patients who progress rapidly during first-line treatment, additional benefit from further cytokine treatment is unlikely. Further studies are needed to see whether crossing over from one cytokine to another is able to increase survival in selected patients who have experienced a long period of stabilization or have relapsed after an initial response.

Other Cytokines

Several other interleukins (for example IL-1, -4, and -6) have been tested in phase I and II trials in renal cell carcinoma, but antitumor activity has been low, with response rates of less than 5%. One of the more promising new agents is IL-12, which promotes cell-mediated immunity through its regulatory effects on T and natural killer (NK) cells. In a randomized phase II trial of IL-12 versus IFN-α in advanced renal cell carcinoma, 30 patients were treated with IL-12 and 2 (7%) achieved a partial response, whereas no responses were seen in the IFN-α arm [52].

Although the activity of IL-12 alone appears low, animal models have noted a synergy between IL-2 and IL-12. This interaction has been shown in a study that assessed in vivo stimulation of IL-12 secretion by subcutaneous low-dose IL-2 in metastatic renal cell carcinoma [53]. By evaluating IL-12 variations in relation to clinical response, a marked significant increase in IL-12 values occurred in patients with disease response or stabilization of disease, whereas progressing patients showed a significant decline in IL-12 levels during IL-2 administration. Thus, IL-2 may stimulate release of IL-12, and this is possibly associated with a favorable prognosis. Further studies of IL-12 as part of combination therapy with IL-2 are needed to see if this synergy can be exploited.

Biochemotherapy

The lack of cross-resistance, nonoverlapping toxicity, and potential synergy between chemotherapy and biological therapy has led to several trials combining cytokines and chemotherapeutic agents (so-called biochemotherapy) in metastatic renal cell carcinoma. One rationale for this approach is that by causing cytotoxicity chemotherapy will release tumor antigens, which are processed by IFN-α–stimulated antigen-presenting cells that in turn activate IL-2–stimulated CTLs. The counterargument would be that chemotherapy may downregulate immunological responses.

A phase III study involving 160 patients has compared IFN-α plus vinblastine (VLB) with vinblastine alone [54]. This study showed a significant benefit for biochemotherapy both in terms of median survival (IFN-α + VLB: 67.6 weeks; VLB: 37.8 weeks; p = .0049) and response rate (IFN-α + VLB: 16.5%; VLB: 2.5%; p = .0025). The increase in survival is both clinically and statistically significant, and long-term survivors who remained in remission after 4 to 5 years were noted.

This study did not address the role of vinblastine in the combination, and it could be argued that the benefit seen is solely due to IFN-α. A phase III study by Fossa and colleagues [55] compared IFN-α with or without vinblastine. They found no statistically significant differences in activity or survival between the two regimens, although combination treatment was associated with a higher response rate (24% versus 11%) and a trend to longer median survival (55 versus 47 weeks). The role of vinblastine in combination with cytokines requires further investigation; it may contribute only modestly to antitumor activity.

The most extensively studied chemotherapeutic agent used in combination with cytokines in the treatment of renal cell carcinoma is 5-fluorouracil (5-FU). The administration of IFN-α with 5-FU modulates the effects of 5-FU, resulting in synergy due to the blocking of thymidine incorporation into DNA. Although in vitro models demonstrated augmentation of cytotoxicity, this was not reflected in the results of a phase II trial where there were no objective clinical responses when IFN-α and 5-FU were given to patients and median survival was only 5 months [56].

The highest response rates in metastatic renal cell carcinoma are obtained using a combination of IFN-α, IL-2, and 5-FU (bolus). This was first described by Atzpodien and colleagues [57] and is an outpatient-based regimen of subcutaneous IFN-α, IL-2, and bolus intravenous 5-FU. Their initial study demonstrated a response rate of 48.6% (four CR and 13 PR out of 35 patients). They went on to confirm the activity of this regimen in a randomized trial comparing IFN-α, IL-2, and 5-FU with oral tamoxifen [58]. There was a response rate of 39% in the IFN-α, IL-2, and 5-FU arm, whereas no responses occurred in patients treated with tamoxifen. Furthermore, overall and progression-free survivals were both significantly improved in the biochemotherapy arm (overall survival: IFN-α, IL-2, and 5-FU median not reached after 42 months versus 14 months for tamoxifen; p < .04; progression-free survival: 13 vs. 4 months, p < .01).

Several other groups have tested this combination and response rates vary widely (Table 7.5). This is probably due to differences in patient characteristics between study groups and/or altered dose intensity and scheduling of the drugs [59–63]. A study by Ravaud and colleagues [64], which gave a response rate of only 1.8%, highlights the second of these points. In their study the dose and scheduling of all three agents differed from that used by Atzpodien et al. [57], and the result suggests that scheduling of cytokines, perhaps particularly in the context of 5-FU, may be important.

The importance of dose, schedule, and patient selection is again shown in a study from the Groupe Francais d'Immunotherapie [65]. Here Negrier and colleagues randomized 131 patients with metastatic renal cell carcinoma to receive subcutaneous IL-2 and IFN-α with or without 5-FU. The dose and schedule was the same as that used by Ravaud and colleagues. There was one PR in the IL-2 and IFN-α arm and five PRs in the IL-2, IFN-α, and 5-FU arm ($p = .1$). Overall survival rates at 1 year were 53% in the IL-2 and IFN-α arm and 52% in the IL-2, IFN-α, and 5-FU arm.

The optimal method of scheduling and delivery of these agents has yet to be established. Our group has explored an alternative way of delivering 5-FU within this combination. 5- Fluorouracil is principally active in the S phase of the cell cycle, and this may be more effective when given as a protracted venous infusion

Table 7.5. Treatment of renal cell carcinoma with interferon-α (IFN-α) + interleukin-2 (IL-2) + 5-fluorouracil (5-FU)

Author, year [reference]	No. of patients	Response rate (%)	Median survival
Atzpodien 1993 [57]	35	49	Not reported
Hofmockel 1996 [59]	34	38	Not reported
Joffe 1996 [60]	55	16	12 months
Ellerhorst 1997 [61]	55	31	23 months
Ravaud 1998 [64]	111	2	12 months
Tourani 1998 [62]	62	19	33% at 2 years
Allen 2000 [68]	55	31	10.7 months
Elias 2000 [63]	38	11	Not reported
Atzpodien 2001 [58]	41	39.1	2.1

(PVI). Protracted venous infusion 5-FU– containing regimens have given high response rates in neoadjuvant treatment of breast cancer [66] and relapsed ovarian cancer [67]. Our study using IFN-α, IL-2, and 5-FU (PVI) showed an overall response rate of 31% in 55 patients (CR: three patients; PR: 14 patients) [68]. Interestingly, there was a trend toward higher response rates and longer survival in the poorer prognosis group, although this did not reach statistical significance. Again this supports the inclusion of fit patients even if they have poor prognostic features in future studies.

Despite high response rates seen with the IFN-α, IL-2, and 5-FU combination, the majority of patients relapse. The concept of continuing immune stimulation in responders is an attractive one and our own group and Atzpodien's are investigating the feasibility of this approach.

Capecitabine, which as stated earlier is selectively activated to 5-FU, has been substituted for 5-FU in this regimen. Atzpodien's group [69] used oral capecitabine with subcutaneous IFN-α and IL-2 and oral 13-cis-retinoic acid to treat 30 patients with metastatic renal cell carcinoma. There were two complete responses and eight partial responses for an overall response rate of 33%. These results are comparable to other 5-FU–based biochemotherapy regimens, with the advantage of oral administration of capecitabine and low toxicity. Without randomized data the contribution of capecitabine and its potential improvement in toxicity cannot be assessed and so Atzpodien's group has initiated a phase III study to investigate its role.

Adjuvant Therapy

The only curative treatment for renal cell carcinoma is complete surgical excision of the primary lesion. As stated earlier, 20% to 30% of patients who initially present with localized disease subsequently relapse after nephrectomy, usually with metastatic disease . Thus there is a need for an effective adjuvant therapy.

Three large randomized trials totaling 250 patients have compared adjuvant interferon with observation in resected Robson stages II (perinephric fat involved) and III (tumor extension into renal vein or inferior vena cava; resected lymph node metastases) [70–72]. None of these studies showed an improvement in survival for adjuvant interferon over observation.

The role of adjuvant high-dose bolus IL-2 for patients with high-risk renal cell carcinoma has recently been addressed in a randomized trial [73]. The authors randomized patients with locally advanced (T3b–4 or N1–3) or postmetastasectomy to one course of high-dose IL-2 or to observation. The study was designed and powered to show an improvement in predicted 2-year disease-free survival from 40% in the observation group to 70% in the treatment group. The accrual goal was 68 patients with locally advanced disease, with 34 patients per treatment arm. Patients who underwent metastasectomy were to be analyzed separately because of their different natural history.

Sixty-nine patients were entered into the study, 44 with locally advanced disease and 25 postmetastasectomy. The study was closed early when an interim analysis determined that the 30% improvement in 2-year disease-free survival could not be achieved despite full accrual. Sixteen of the 21 locally advanced patients receiving IL-2 relapsed compared with 15 of 23 in the observation arm ($p = .73$). Extension of the analysis to include metastasectomy patients made no difference in disease-free survival or overall survival. As the authors concede, a study powered for an improvement in disease-free survival as large as 30% was highly ambitious, considering that high-dose IL-2 is associated with an objective overall response rate of only 15% to 20% in good performance status patients with advanced renal cell carcinoma.

The high response rates seen with the IFN-α, IL-2, and 5-FU combination in metastatic disease has led the EORTC to undertake a randomized trial to assess whether a single cycle of biochemotherapy (IFN-α, IL-2, and 5-FU) is beneficial after resection of high-risk renal cell carcinoma. Standard therapy for fully resected renal cell carcinoma outside of clinical trials remains observation.

Angiogenesis Inhibitors

Angiogenesis is the growth of new microvessels. The growth of tumors beyond 1 to 2 mm^3 depends on angiogenesis, which is necessary for the supply of nutrients and also provides a route for metastasis. In adults the vascular endothelium is a quiescent tissue with a low cell division rate, and thus pathological angiogenesis must occur to allow tumor development. A number of proangiogenic factors (e.g., basic fibroblast growth factor and vascular endothelial growth factor [VEGF]) have been identified, as well as antiangiogenic factors (e.g., angiostatin and endostatin). The balance between these factors is important in tumor dormancy and control of micrometastases, where the apoptotic rate remains high until angiogenesis occurs. This shift in balance is termed the "angiogenic switch," which is a complex process resulting in a shift in the balance between stimulators and inhibitors of angiogenesis, during which inhibitors are downregulated [74].

Neovascularization provides not only a perfusion stimulus for tumor growth, but also a paracrine effect, which results from endothelial-derived growth factors and cytokines that stimulate growth and migration of tumor cells. This paracrine effect is thought to operate in both directions; that is, endothelial cell survival and growth are driven by tumor-derived endothelial factors. This two-cell compartment model of tumor growth may influence the design of clinical trials; for instance, angiogenesis inhibitors can be combined with conventional cytotoxic therapy.

The close relationship between angiogenesis and tumor growth and metastasis make it an attractive target for cancer therapy. Also the amplification factor seen in the relationship between tumor and vascular endothelial cells means that suppression of one endothelial cell could inhibit the growth of approximately 100 tumor cells [75]. Initial experience with angiogenesis inhibitors in animal models and from early clinical trials in advanced cancer has led to general guidelines about their use [74]:

1. Long-term therapy is necessary. Antiangiogenic therapy is a relatively slower process than cytotoxic therapy.

2. Antiangiogenic therapy should not be interrupted because of the ability of microvessels to regrow quickly.

3. Resistance does not appear to be a problem with long-term use. The theoretical basis for this is that endothelial cells, unlike tumor cells, are not considered to be mutating and thus are unlikely to generate resistant clones.

4. Combination of antioangiogenic agents with different mechanisms of action and/or with cytotoxic agents appears to be more effective [76]. Such combinations in animal models have been curative, whereas either agent alone is merely inhibitory [77].

Angiogenesis Inhibitors Used in Clinical Trials to Treat Renal Cell Carcinoma

TNP-470 is a fumagillin analogue and is one of the first angiogenesis inhibitors to undergo clinical testing. Fumagillin was originally isolated from *Aspergillus fumigatus* contaminating endothelial cell cultures [78] and is a potent inhibitor of endothelial growth in vitro and in vivo. A number of analogues of fumagillin were synthesized, and TNP-470 was selected as the least toxic compound with the greatest antiangiogenic effect [78].

A phase II trial of TNP-470 was carried out in 33 patients with metastatic renal cell carcinoma [79]. There was only one partial response of short duration (response rate 3%), but six patients (18%) had stabilization of disease for 6 months or longer. At a median follow-up of 14 months, median survival is 56 weeks. Therapy was reasonably tolerated, although neurocortical toxicities were common (67% of patients) and led to withdrawal of five patients. Fatigue and asthenia were also common and were seen in 60% of patients.

This patient group had been heavily pretreated, and it is unclear whether this resulted in accrual of patients with indolent disease (median interval from diagnosis of metastatic disease to study initiation was 14 months). Thus, was the prolonged overall and progression-free survival in several patients due to TNP-470, or was it merely a reflection of the natural history of their disease? Further studies using TNP-470 are warranted, and combination with other angiogenesis inhibitors, cytotoxic drugs, and cytokines is indicated.

An attractive option would be the combination of TNP-470 with IFN-α, which is known to have both antiangiogenic and direct antitumor activity. Future studies should also address ways of increasing exposure to TNP-470, which animal studies suggest is necessary to maximize its antiangiogenic properties. In this study exposure was likely to be suboptimal, as the half-life of TNP-470 and its active metabolite are only 2 and 6 minutes, respectively. It may also be that the greatest benefit in using TNP-470 and other antiangiogenics to delay progression in renal cell carcinoma is seen in the adjuvant or minimal disease setting.

The likelihood of successfully introducing a new drug increases when the mechanisms of both the drug and the disease are well understood and linked in a biologically coherent fashion.

This has been shown to a degree by the use of bevacizumab in the treatment of metastatic renal cancer. Studies of the hereditary form of clear-cell renal carcinoma, which occurs in the von Hippel–Lindau tumor syndrome, led to the identification of the von Hippel–Lindau tumor-suppressor gene *(VHL)* [80]. An inactivated *VHL* gene inherited from either parent causes von Hippel–Lindau disease, in which tumors with multiple blood vessels develop in the central nervous system and the risk of clear cell carcinoma of the kidney is increased. The development of tumors in von Hippel–Lindau disease is linked to loss of the remaining normal *VHL* allele, thus eliminating the *VHL* gene product. The gene is also mutated in most sporadic cases of clear cell renal carcinoma, where both alleles have acquired mutations or deletions [80]. Tumors caused by the inactivation of the *VHL* tumor-suppressor gene should be an ideal testing ground for VEGF inhibition because there is a close relationship between *VHL* inactivation and VEGF overproduction through a mechanism involving hypoxia-inducible factor α.

Bevacizumab is a humanized version of a murine monoclonal antibody against VEGF. Yang and colleagues [81] conducted a randomized phase II trial comparing placebo with bevacizumab at low or high dose in patients with metastatic clear cell renal carcinoma. The trial was stopped after the interim analysis met the criteria for early stopping based on the difference in time to progression between the placebo and high-dose bevacizumab arms. A total of 116 patients were randomly assigned to placebo (40 patients), low-dose bevacizumab (37 patients), or high-dose bevacizumab (39 patients). There was a significant prolongation of the time to progression in the high-dose antibody group as compared to placebo (hazard ratio 2.55; $p < .001$). The probability of being progression-free for patients given high-dose antibody, low-dose antibody, or placebo was 64%, 39%, and 20%, respectively, at 4 months and 30%, 14%, and 5% at 8 months. Only four patients achieved objective responses (all partial responses), all of whom received high-dose bevacizumab. Thus the response rate for high-dose antibody was 10%. There were no significant differences in survival between the treatment groups. However, time to disease progression and overall response rate were the primary end points. Survival was a secondary end point, as patients whose disease progressed on placebo were offered crossover to either low-dose bevacizumab or low-dose bevacizumab and thalidomide.

There were no significant associations between detectable pre-treatment levels of VEGF and clinical response or time to progression in either bevacizumab group. However, the authors note the limited sensitivity of the assay used. After antibody treatment is started, plasma levels of VEGF are difficult to interpret, as the assay measures both free and antibody-bound VEGF, but the levels rose steadily. This study is encouraging and could serve as a platform for the integration of antioangiogenic agents into the treatment of renal cell cancer. Phase III studies are needed to address the true clinical benefits of VEGF inhibition. A crucial question is whether status of expression of the *VHL* gene product affects response to treatment. Knowledge of the function of the *VHL* gene product and its intimate association with hypoxia-inducible factor α support combination with agents that interrupt other hypoxia-inducible genes such as platelet-derived growth factor.

Several other antiangiogenic agents have shown potential activity in phase I/II trials, some of which are discussed below.

Vascular endothelial growth factor (VEGF) is abnormally expressed in up to 70% of renal cell carcinomas and is thus a rational therapeutic target. SU5416 inhibits VEGF-mediated signaling through Flk-1, a transmembrane tyrosine kinase, resulting in decreased angiogenesis. In a phase I trial of 63 patients, stabilization of disease for greater than 6 months was seen in several tumor types including renal cell carcinoma [82]. A recent study assessed the activity of SU5416 in 29 patients with renal cell carcinoma. A low response rate was seen with one minor response and five patients achieving stable disease (3 months or longer) [83].

AE-941 (Neovastat) is a naturally occurring product extracted from cartilage that has antiangiogenic properties [84]. It inhibits several steps of the angiogenesis process, including matrix metalloproteinase activities and VEGF signaling pathways. Also, AE-941 induces endothelial cell apoptosis and tissue-type plasminogen activator activity, suggesting that it is a multifunctional antiangiogenic drug. Twenty-two patients with refractory renal cell carcinoma were treated as part of a larger phase II study assessing two dosing levels of neovastat [85]. Median survival time was significantly longer (16.3 versus 7.1 months; $p = .01$) in patients treated with Neovastat 240 mL/day ($n = 14$) compared with patients receiving 60 mL/day ($n = 8$). This difference in survival was not explained by any significant differences in major prognostic factors between the two groups. Neovastat is administered orally and has low toxicity. It is now being evaluated in a phase III trial in patients who have failed immunotherapy.

There is currently considerable interest in antiangiogenesis, with several new agents in development, many of which have entered clinical trials. Two of the most interesting compounds are angiostatin and endostatin, both of which were isolated by Folkman and colleagues. Angiostatin is a proteolytic degradation product of plasminogen and is a specific inhibitor of endothelial proliferation [86]. It is the first angiogenesis inhibitor that can cause regression of human cancer xenografts in mice. A microscopic dormant state in which virtually all neovascularization has been blocked is achieved by prolonged blockade of angiogenesis [87].

Endostatin, a proteolytic degradation product of collagen type XVIII, has also been shown to cause tumor regression in murine carcinoma models. Tumors recurred when treatment was stopped but regressed again when endostatin therapy was recommenced. Interestingly, when therapy was withdrawn for a second time, no tumor recurrence was observed [88]. Both angiostatin and endostatin have entered clinical trials that will determine their efficacy. Initial phase I trials with endostatin have shown it is well tolerated when treating several malignancies, but little clinical activity has been demonstrated [89].

The integration of antioangiogenic drugs into current practice may represent an important advance. New therapeutic end points, such as disease stabilization, may be required during the evaluation of these compounds. Imaging techniques, such as Doppler (measuring blood flow) and positron emission tomography (PET) scanning (measuring tumor metabolism) may aid in assessing response to antioangiogenic treatment. Other useful indicators of response may be angiogenic factors such as VEGF and fibroblast growth factor (FGF) in plasma and urine.

Thalidomide

Thalidomide has been discovered to have powerful antiangiogenic activity. Its mechanism of action is complex including breakdown of messenger RNA (mRNA) of a number of molecules such as FGF and tumor necrosis factor-α (TNF-α). Our group's phase II study tested low-dose thalidomide (100 mg orally every night) in 66 patients with metastatic cancer, including several with renal cell carcinoma [90]. There were three partial responses and 13 stabilizations of previously progressive disease (3 for more than 3 months) in the 18 patients with renal cell carcinoma who were treated. Treatment was well tolerated and no World Health Organization (WHO) grade 3 or 4 toxicities were seen. The main toxicity was lethargy (38 patients grade 1, eight patients grade 2), but conversely, several patients experienced improvement in sleep and appetite. In a further study using thalidomide, 600 mg orally every night, there were two partial responses. Seven patients had stable disease for greater than 6 months and five had stable disease for between 3 and 6 months out of the 25 patients treated [91]. In patients who achieved a partial response or who had stable disease for at least 3 months. a statistically significant decrease in serum TNF-α levels was seen ($p = .05$).

Several other groups have now published studies of thalidomide in renal cell carcinoma. Overall response rate in these trials was 6%. with 10 partial responses out of 158 patients [90–95]. The low response rates do not support the use of thalidomide to induce responses in patients with metastatic renal cell carcinoma. However, its actions may only be able to achieve disease stabilization by cytostatic inhibition of further tumor growth, and so this may be a more appropriate treatment end point than objective responses. Stabilization of disease is recognized as part of the natural history of renal cell carcinoma, although this is unlikely to occur in patients who have progressed through cytokine therapy. To address whether thalidomide can extend time to progression and improve survival, a phase III randomized trial has been initiated by ECOG that compares low-dose interferon with or without thalidomide.

The exact mechanism of action of thalidomide is unknown and this requires further investigation. A possible mechanism in renal cell carcinoma is inhibition of TNF-α, which is known to be secreted by renal cell carcinomas. This cytokine enhances neoangiogenesis and stimulation of renal carcinoma cells by IL-6, and contributes to many systemic features of advanced malignancy, for example, cachexia and malaise. Two new classes of thalidomide have been developed: one class of compounds are potent phosphodiesterase 4 inhibitors that inhibit TNF-α but have little effect on T-cell activation [96]. The other class of compounds, similar to thalidomide, are not phosphodiesterase 4 inhibitors, but inhibit TNF-α and IL-6, and stimulate T-cell proliferation and IL-2 and IFN-γ production. One of the new immunomodulatory analogues, CC-5013, has shown impressive activity in refractory multiple myeloma [97]. The use of these novel compounds will help to elucidate the mechanisms that underlie thalidomide's activity in renal cell carcinoma.

The combination of thalidomide with immunotherapy is an attractive one. Our group commenced a phase II study of IFN-α (9 MU 3 times/week subcutaneously) and thalidomide (400 mg). Unfortunately, unexpected neurological toxicity was seen in four of 13 patients treated with this regimen and the study has been closed [98]. The authors recommended that caution be used when combining these agents and lower doses of IFN-α.

A recent study has confirmed the feasibility of combining thalidomide with lower doses of IFN-α [99]. Thirty patients were given IFN-α (0.9 MU 3 times/day subcutaneously for 1 month and subsequently 1.2 MU 3 times/day) and thalidomide (100 mg/day for 1 week and 300 mg/day thereafter). The response rate was 20%, all responses were partial, and median survival was 14.9 months. The most common toxicity was sensory neuropathy, causing 19 patients (63%) to discontinue thalidomide. Median duration of thalidomide treatment was 6.5 months and that of IFN-α was 7.2 months. Interestingly, serum VEGF levels decreased more in patients who responded to therapy compared to those who had stable or progressive disease ($p = .036$). This combination is undoubtedly neurotoxic, and careful follow-up of patients is needed. Results of an ongoing ECOG phase III trial comparing IFN-α with or without thalidomide are awaited with interest.

The combination of thalidomide with IL-2 has also been addressed in a recent phase II study [100]. Out of 37 patients there was one complete response, 14 partial responses, and 11 patients with stable disease. Time on therapy ranged from 3 to 15 months. Twenty-six patients continue on therapy with either objective response or stable disease. Treatment was generally well tolerated with mainly grade 1 to 2 toxicities. This therefore appears to be a promising new regimen, and a phase III trial of IL-2 plus thalidomide versus IL-2 versus thalidomide is planned.

Conclusion

Patients with metastatic renal cell still have a very poor prognosis and there remains the continued need for research. It should be noted that patients entering clinical trials are often highly selected, particularly where protocols of intensive treatments are involved. Entry criteria to most studies are often those that predict response and good survival, such as good performance status and nephrectomy. Results therefore may not be applicable to an unselected population of patients.

It is important to remember that many of the treatments discussed here are still in their infancy, compared to conventional cancer treatments. It is likely that over the next few years some of these therapies will become important management options. Of the newer agents, cytokines have been shown to improve overall survival as demonstrated by three randomized controlled studies.

Our knowledge of the molecular biology of renal cell carcinoma is ever increasing, allowing new therapeutic options such as signal transduction inhibitors, antiangiogenesis agents, tumor vaccines, dendritic cell vaccines, monoclonal antibodies, antisense oligonucleotides, and gene therapy to be developed. The translation of targeted biological therapy into a front-line treatment, as exemplified by the use of trastuzumab in breast cancer, remains the ultimate goal for future trials.

Other aims include:

- The identification of patients most likely to respond to treatment
- The development of methods to maintain response
- A decrease in the toxicity of treatment
- Integration of new agents into currently active regimens

Whenever possible patients undergoing systemic treatment should be entered into appropriate clinical trials. Standard therapy for fit patients is single-agent interferon-α or single-agent interleukin-2.

Controversies and Outstanding Issues

1. Can we establish any benefit for adjuvant cytokine therapy?
2. Is there a role for adjuvant kinase inhibitors?
3. Can we select patients for treatment on the basis of biological markers?

References

1. Jemal A, et al. Cancer statistics, 2002. CA Cancer J Clin 2002;52(1):23–47.
2. Motzer RJ, Bander NH, Nanus DM. Renal-cell carcinoma. N Engl J Med 1996;335(12):865–875.
3. Dhote R, et al. Risk factors for adult renal cell carcinoma: a systematic review and implications for prevention. BJU Int 2000; 86(1):20–27.
4. Yagoda A, Abi-Rached B, Petrylak D. Chemotherapy for advanced renal-cell carcinoma: 1983–1993. Semin Oncol 1995;22(1):42–60.
5. Elson PJ, Witte RS, Trump DL. Prognostic factors for survival in patients with recurrent or metastatic renal cell carcinoma. Cancer Res 1988;48(24 pt 1):7310–7313.
6. Palmer PA, et al. Prognostic factors for survival in patients with advanced renal cell carcinoma treated with recombinant interleukin-2. Ann Oncol 1992;3(6):475–480.
7. Jones M, et al. The impact of interleukin-2 on survival in renal cancer: a multivariate analysis. Cancer Biother 1993;8(4):275–288.
8. Fossa SD, Kramar A, Droz JP. Prognostic factors and survival in patients with metastatic renal cell carcinoma treated with chemotherapy or interferon-alpha. Eur J Cancer 1994;30A(9):1310–1314.
9. Motzer RJ, et al. Survival and prognostic stratification of 670 patients with advanced renal cell carcinoma. J Clin Oncol 1999; 17(8):2530–2540.
10. Motzer RJ, et al. Prognostic factors for survival in previously treated patients with metastatic renal cell carcinoma. J Clin Oncol 2004;22(3):454–463.
11. Motzer RJ, et al. Treatment outcome and survival associated with metastatic renal cell carcinoma of non-clear-cell histology. J Clin Oncol 2002;20(9):2376–2381.
12. Kudoh S, et al. Defective granzyme B gene expression and lytic response in T lymphocytes infiltrating human renal cell carcinoma. J Immunother 1997;20(6):479–487.
13. Ulchaker J, et al. Interferon-gamma production by T lymphocytes from renal cell carcinoma patients: evidence of impaired secretion in response to interleukin-12. J Immunother 1999;22(1): 71–79.
14. Almand B, et al. Increased production of immature myeloid cells in cancer patients: a mechanism of immunosuppression in cancer. J Immunol 2001;166(1):678–689.
15. Finke JH, et al. Tumor-infiltrating lymphocytes in patients with renal-cell carcinoma. Ann N Y Acad Sci 1988;532:387–394.

16. Van Den Eynde BJ, et al. A new antigen recognized by cytolytic T lymphocytes on a human kidney tumor results from reverse strand transcription. J Exp Med 1999;190(12):1793–1800.

17. Motzer RJ, et al. Effect of cytokine therapy on survival for patients with advanced renal cell carcinoma. J Clin Oncol 2000;18(9): 1928–1935.

18. Negrier S, et al. Prognostic factors of survival and rapid progression in 782 patients with metastatic renal carcinomas treated by cytokines: a report from the Groupe Francais d'Immunotherapie. Ann Oncol 2002;13(9):1460–1468.

19. Van Poppel H, Baert L. Nephrectomy for metastatic renal cell carcinoma and surgery for distant metastases. Acta Urol Belg 1996;64(2):11–17.

20. Piltz S, et al. Long-term results after pulmonary resection of renal cell carcinoma metastases. Ann Thorac Surg 2002;73(4):1082–1087.

21. Le Francois D, et al. Evolution of cell-mediated immunity in mice bearing tumors produced by a mammary carcinoma cell line. Influence of tumor growth, surgical removal, and treatment with irradiated tumor cells. J Natl Cancer Inst 1971;46(5):981–987.

22. Whitney RB, Levy JG, Smith AG. Influence of tumor size and surgical resection on cell-mediated immunity in mice. J Natl Cancer Inst 1974;53(1):111–116.

23. Dadian G, et al. Immunological parameters in peripheral blood of patients with renal cell carcinoma before and after nephrectomy. Br J Urol 1994;74(1):15–22.

24. Pantuck AZA, Shvarts O, Gitlitz B, deKernion J, Figlin R, Belldegrun A. Natural history and the role of nephrectomy in the biology of RCC: the UCLA experience. Proc Am Soc Clin Oncol 2000;19:1348.

25. Flanigan RC, et al. Nephrectomy followed by interferon alfa-2b compared with interferon alfa-2b alone for metastatic renal-cell cancer. N Engl J Med 2001;345(23):1655–1659.

26. Mickisch GH, et al. Radical nephrectomy plus interferon-alfa-based immunotherapy compared with interferon alfa alone in metastatic renal-cell carcinoma: a randomised trial. Lancet 2001;358(9286): 966–970.

27. Flanigan RC, et al. Cytoreductive nephrectomy in patients with metastatic renal cancer: a combined analysis. J Urol 2004;171(3): 1071–1076.

28. Naitoh J, et al. Metastatic renal cell carcinoma with concurrent inferior vena caval invasion: long-term survival after combination therapy with radical nephrectomy, vena caval thrombectomy and postoperative immunotherapy. J Urol 1999;162(1):46–50.

29. Lineham WM, et al. Cancer of the kidney and ureter. In: Devita VT, ed. Cancer: Principles and Practice of Oncology. Philadephia: Lippincott Williams and Wilkins, 1997:1271–1300.

30. Motzer RJ, et al. Phase II trial of branched peg interferon-alpha 2a (40 kDa) for patients with advanced renal cell carcinoma. Ann Oncol 2002;13(11):1799–1805.

31. Bukowski, R, et al. Pegylated interferon alfa-2b treatment for patients with solid tumors: a phase I/II study. J Clin Oncol 2002; 20(18):3841–3849.

32. Interferon-alpha and survival in metastatic renal carcinoma: early results of a randomised controlled trial. Medical Research Council Renal Cancer Collaborators. Lancet 1999;353(9146):14–17.

33. Hancock B, Griffiths G, Ritchie A, et al., on behalf of the MRC Renal Cancer Collaborators. Updated results of the MRC randomised controlled trial of alpha interferon vs. MPA in patients with metastatic renal carcinoma. Proc Am Soc Clin Oncol 2000;abstract 1336.

34. Coppin C, et al. Immunotherapy for advanced renal cell cancer. Cochrane Database Syst Rev 2000(3):CD001425.

35. Hoffman AD, et al. Expression of retinoic acid receptor beta in human renal cell carcinomas correlates with sensitivity to the antiproliferative effects of 13–cis-retinoic acid. Clin Cancer Res 1996;2(6):1077–1082.

36. Motzer RJ, et al. Interferon alfa-2a and 13–cis-retinoic acid in renal cell carcinoma: antitumor activity in a phase II trial and interactions in vitro. J Clin Oncol 1995;13(8):1950–1957.

37. Motzer RJ, et al. Phase III trial of interferon alfa-2a with or without 13–cis-retinoic acid for patients with advanced renal cell carcinoma. J Clin Oncol 2000;18(16):2972–2980.

38. Gleave ME, et al. Interferon gamma-1b compared with placebo in metastatic renal-cell carcinoma. Canadian Urologic Oncology Group. N Engl J Med 1998;338(18):1265–1271.

39. De Mulder PH, et al. EORTC (30885) randomised phase III study with recombinant interferon alpha and recombinant interferon alpha and gamma in patients with advanced renal cell carcinoma. The EORTC Genitourinary Group. Br J Cancer 1995;71(2):371–375.

40. Fyfe G, et al. Results of treatment of 255 patients with metastatic renal cell carcinoma who received high-dose recombinant interleukin-2 therapy. J Clin Oncol 1995;13(3):688–696.

41. Fisher RI, Rosenberg SA, Fyfe G. Long-term survival update for high-dose recombinant interleukin-2 in patients with renal cell carcinoma. Cancer J Sci Am 2000;6(suppl 1):S55–57.

42. Yang JC, et al. Randomized comparison of high-dose and low-dose intravenous interleukin-2 for the therapy of metastatic renal cell carcinoma: an interim report. J Clin Oncol 1994;12(8):1572–1576.

43. Yang JC, et al. Randomized study of high-dose and low-dose interleukin-2 in patients with metastatic renal cancer. J Clin Oncol 2003;21(16):3127–3132.

44. Bukowski RM. Natural history and therapy of metastatic renal cell carcinoma: the role of interleukin-2. Cancer 1997;80(7):1198–1220.

45. Lindsey KR, Rosenberg SA, Sherry RM. Impact of the number of treatment courses on the clinical response of patients who receive high-dose bolus interleukin-2. J Clin Oncol 2000;18(9):1954–1959.

46. Rosenberg SA, et al. Prospective randomized trial of high-dose interleukin-2 alone or in conjunction with lymphokine-activated killer cells for the treatment of patients with advanced cancer. J Natl Cancer Inst 1993;85(8):622–632.

47. Figlin RA, et al. Treatment of metastatic renal cell carcinoma with nephrectomy, interleukin-2 and cytokine-primed or CD8(+) selected tumor infiltrating lymphocytes from primary tumor. J Urol 1997;158(3 Pt 1):740–745.

48. Figlin RA, et al. Multicenter, randomized, phase III trial of CD8(+) tumor-infiltrating lymphocytes in combination with recombinant interleukin-2 in metastatic renal cell carcinoma. J Clin Oncol 1999;17(8):2521–2529.

49. Sherry RM, Rosenberg SA, Yang JC. Relapse after response to interleukin-2–based immunotherapy: patterns of progression and response to retreatment. J Immunother 1991;10(5):371–375.

50. Negrier S, et al. Recombinant human interleukin-2, recombinant human interferon alfa-2a, or both in metastatic renal-cell carcinoma. Groupe Francais d'Immunotherapie. N Engl J Med 1998;338(18):1272–1278.

51. Escudier B, et al. Cytokines in metastatic renal cell carcinoma: is it useful to switch to interleukin-2 or interferon after failure of a first treatment? Groupe Francais d'Immunotherape. J Clin Oncol 1999;17(7):2039–2043.

52. Motzer RJ, et al. Randomized multicenter phase II trial of subcutaneous recombinant human interleukin-12 versus interferon-alpha 2a for patients with advanced renal cell carcinoma. J Interferon Cytokine Res 2001;21(4):257–263.

53. Lissoni P, et al. In vivo stimulation of IL-12 secretion by subcutaneous low-dose IL-2 in metastatic cancer patients. Br J Cancer 1998;77(11):1957–1960.

54. Pyrhonen S, et al. Prospective randomized trial of interferon alfa-2a plus vinblastine versus vinblastine alone in patients with advanced renal cell cancer. J Clin Oncol 1999;17(9):2859–2867.

55. Fossa SD, et al. Recombinant interferon alfa-2a with or without vinblastine in metastatic renal cell carcinoma: results of a European multi-center phase III study. Ann Oncol 1992;3(4):301–305.

56. Murphy BR, et al. A phase II trial of interferon alpha-2A plus fluorouracil in advanced renal cell carcinoma. A Hoosier Oncology Group study. Invest New Drugs 1992;10(3):225–230.

57. Atzpodien J, et al. Interleukin-2 in combination with interferon-alpha and 5–fluorouracil for metastatic renal cell cancer. Eur J Cancer 1993;29A(suppl 5):S6–8.

58. Atzpodien J, et al. IL-2 in combination with IFN- alpha and 5–FU versus tamoxifen in metastatic renal cell carcinoma: long-term results of a controlled randomized clinical trial. Br J Cancer 2001;85(8):1130–1136.

59. Hofmockel G, et al. Immunochemotherapy for metastatic renal cell carcinoma using a regimen of interleukin-2, interferon-alpha and 5– fluorouracil. J Urol 1996;156(1):18–21.

60. Joffe JK, et al. A phase II study of interferon-alpha, interleukin-2 and 5–fluorouracil in advanced renal carcinoma: clinical data and laboratory evidence of protease activation. Br J Urol 1996;77(5): 638–649.

61. Ellerhorst JA, et al. Phase II trial of 5– fluorouracil, interferon-alpha and continuous infusion interleukin-2 for patients with metastatic renal cell carcinoma. Cancer 1997;80(11):2128–2132.

62. Tourani JM, et al. Outpatient treatment with subcutaneous interleukin-2 and interferon alfa administration in combination with fluorouracil in patients with metastatic renal cell carcinoma: results of a sequential nonrandomized phase II study. Subcutaneous Administration Proleukin Program Cooperative Group. J Clin Oncol 1998;16(7):2505–2513.

63. Elias L, et al. Infusional interleukin-2 and 5–fluorouracil with subcutaneous interferon-alpha for the treatment of patients with advanced renal cell carcinoma: a southwest oncology group Phase II study. Cancer 2000;89(3):597–603.

64. Ravaud A, et al. Subcutaneous interleukin-2, interferon alfa-2a, and continuous infusion of fluorouracil in metastatic renal cell carcinoma: a multicenter phase II trial. Groupe Francais d'Immunotherapie. J Clin Oncol 1998;16(8):2728–2732.

65. Negrier S, et al. Treatment of patients with metastatic renal carcinoma with a combination of subcutaneous interleukin-2 and interferon alfa with or without fluorouracil. Groupe Francais d'Immunotherapie, Federation Nationale des Centres de Lutte Contre le Cancer. J Clin Oncol 2000;18(24):4009–4015.

66. Smith IE, et al. High complete remission rates with primary neoadjuvant infusional chemotherapy for large early breast cancer. J Clin Oncol 1995;13(2):424–429.

67. Ahmed FMP, Macfarlane V, Gore M. Infusional chemotherapy (cisplatin, epirubicin, 5–FU: ECF) for patients with epithelial ovarian carcinoma. In: 9th NCI-EORTC Symposium on New Drug Therapy, 1996, Amsterdam.

68. Allen MJ, et al. Protracted venous infusion 5–fluorouracil in combination with subcutaneous interleukin-2 and alpha-interferon in patients with metastatic renal cell cancer: a phase II study. Br J Cancer 2000;83(8):980–985.

69. Oevermann K, et al. Capecitabine in the treatment of metastatic renal cell carcinoma. Br J Cancer 2000;83(5):583–587.

70. Porzsolt F. Adjuvant therapy of renal cell carcinoma with interferon alpha-2a. Proc Am Soc Clin Oncol 1992;11:622.

71. Trump DL, Elson P, Propert K, et al. Randomized, controlled trial of adjuvant therapy with lymphoblastoid interferon (L-IFN) in resected, high-risk renal cell carcinoma (HR-RCC) Proc Am Soc Clin Oncol 1966;15:253.

72. Pizzocaro G, et al. Interferon adjuvant to radical nephrectomy in Robson stages II and III renal cell carcinoma: a multicentric randomized study. J Clin Oncol 2001;19(2):425–431.

73. Clark JI, et al. Adjuvant high-dose bolus interleukin-2 for patients with high-risk renal cell carcinoma: a cytokine working group randomized trial. J Clin Oncol 2003;21(16):3133–3140.

74. Folkman J. Antiangiogenic therapy. In: Devita VT, ed. Cancer: Principles and Practice of Oncology. Philadephia: Lippincott Williams and Wilkins, 1997.

75. Modzelewski RA, et al. Isolation and identification of fresh tumor-derived endothelial cells from a murine RIF-1 fibrosarcoma. Cancer Res 1994;54(2):336–339.

76. Kato T, et al. Enhanced suppression of tumor growth by combination of angiogenesis inhibitor O-(chloroacetyl-carbamoyl)fumagillol (TNP-470) and cytotoxic agents in mice. Cancer Res 1994;54(19):5143–5147.

77. Teicher BA, et al. Potentiation of cytotoxic cancer therapies by TNP-470 alone and with other anti-angiogenic agents. Int J Cancer 1994;57(6):920–925.

78. Ingber D, et al. Synthetic analogues of fumagillin that inhibit angiogenesis and suppress tumour growth. Nature 1990;348(6301):555–557.

79. Stadler WM, et al. Multi-institutional study of the angiogenesis inhibitor TNP-470 in metastatic renal carcinoma. J Clin Oncol 1999;17(8):2541–2545.

80. George DJ, Kaelin WG Jr. The von Hippel-Lindau protein, vascular endothelial growth factor, and kidney cancer. N Engl J Med 2003;349(5):419–421.

81. Yang JC, et al. A randomized trial of bevacizumab, an anti-vascular endothelial growth factor antibody, for metastatic renal cancer. N Engl J Med 2003;349(5):427–434.

82. Rosen L, Mulay M, Mayers A, et al. Phase I dose- escalating trial of SU5416, a novel angiogenesis inhibitor in patients with advanced malignancies (meeting abstract). Proc Am Soc Clin Oncol 1999;18:618.

83. Kuenen BC, et al. Efficacy and toxicity of the angiogenesis inhibitor SU5416 as a single agent in patients with advanced renal cell carcinoma, melanoma, and soft tissue sarcoma. Clin Cancer Res 2003;9(5):1648–1655.

84. Gingras D, et al. Matrix proteinase inhibition by AE-941, a multifunctional antiangiogenic compound. Anticancer Res 2001;21(1A): 145–155.

85. Batist G, et al. Neovastat (AE-941) in refractory renal cell carcinoma patients: report of a phase II trial with two dose levels. Ann Oncol 2002;13(8):1259–1263.

86. O'Reilly MS, et al. Angiostatin: a novel angiogenesis inhibitor that mediates the suppression of metastases by a Lewis lung carcinoma. Cell 1994;79(2):315–328.

87. O'Reilly MS, et al. Angiostatin induces and sustains dormancy of human primary tumors in mice. Nat Med 1996;2(6):689–692.

88. O'Reilly MS, et al. Endostatin: an endogenous inhibitor of angiogenesis and tumor growth. Cell 1997;88(2):277–285.

89. Herbst RS, et al. Phase I study of recombinant human endostatin in patients with advanced solid tumors. J Clin Oncol 2002;20(18): 3792–3803.

90. Eisen T, et al. Continuous low dose thalidomide: a phase II study in advanced melanoma, renal cell, ovarian and breast cancer. Br J Cancer 2000;82(4):812–817.

91. Stebbing J, et al. The treatment of advanced renal cell cancer with high-dose oral thalidomide. Br J Cancer 2001;85(7):953–958.

92. Motzer RJ, et al. Phase II trial of thalidomide for patients with advanced renal cell carcinoma. J Clin Oncol 2002;20(1):302–306.

93. Minor DR, et al. A phase II study of thalidomide in advanced metastatic renal cell carcinoma. Invest New Drugs 2002;20(4): 389–393.

94. Escudier B, et al. Phase II trial of thalidomide in renal-cell carcinoma. Ann Oncol 2002;13(7):1029–1035.

95. Daliani DD, et al. A pilot study of thalidomide in patients with progressive metastatic renal cell carcinoma. Cancer 2002;95(4): 758–765.

96. Corral LG, et al. Differential cytokine modulation and T cell activation by two distinct classes of thalidomide analogues that are potent inhibitors of TNF-alpha. J Immunol 1999;163(1):380–386.

97. Richardson PG, et al. Immunomodulatory drug CC-5013 overcomes drug resistance and is well tolerated in patients with relapsed multiple myeloma. Blood 2002;100(9):3063–3067.

98. Nathan PD, Gore ME, Eisen TG. Unexpected toxicity of combination thalidomide and interferon alpha-2a treatment in metastatic renal cell carcinoma. J Clin Oncol 2002;20(5):1429–1430.

99. Hernberg M, et al. Interferon alfa-2b three times daily and thalidomide in the treatment of metastatic renal cell carcinoma. J Clin Oncol 2003;21(20):3770–3776.

100. Amato R, Schell J, Thompson N, Moore R, Miles B. Phase II study of thalidomide and interleukin-2 in patients with metastatic renal cell carcinoma. Proc Am Soc Clin Oncol 2003;abstract 1556.

8

Novel Therapies for Renal Cell Cancer

Mayer N. Fishman

Key Points

1. There is now real hope for patients with renal cell cancer because of effective new treatments.
2. Minor response rates are seen with chemotherapy agents.
3. There are major responses to the pan growth factor receptor and angiogenesis inhibitors.
4. Dendritic cell therapy may be effective.
5. Vaccination programs are producing interesting results.

Introduction

The discovery of diverse details of the genetics, cell biology, and pathology of disease and the extensive infrastructure for synthesis and testing of targeted drugs or immune strategies are a basis to be hopeful that innovative, effective, widely applicable therapies can be realized for metastatic kidney cancer. High-dose interleukin-2 had been the sole medical therapy approved by the U.S. Food and Drug Administration (FDA) for the treatment of metastatic renal cancer, and interferon-α, also in widespread use, has had approval in Europe. More than 100 published single-arm/single-drug kidney cancer trials, many based on sound preclinical hypotheses, would seem to be a basis for pessimism. Partial response and disease stabilization at high frequency led to the approval of sorafenib and sunitinib. Whereas progress in conventional cytotoxics has largely bypassed renal cancer, and immune therapies have had dramatic success limited to a minority of patients, some therapies may turn out to be broadly tolerated and efficacious. This is an era for optimism for the application of new technology to kidney cancer therapy.

Looking backward, little seems more precarious than the optimistic projections for clinical trial strategies based on the experience of ex vivo preclinical tests, in vitro testing of cell lines, or murine models. Favorable results of uncontrolled series must be confirmed with randomized testing. The interval from initial safety testing until availability for clinical use routinely exceeds 5 years. Good news of early responders in phase I trials travels fast, along with frustration about the absence of access to drugs in early development. Nonetheless, these preclinical and early-phase trials are a key part of the means by which new compounds or strategies arrive for testing in pivotal clinical trial testing. Much attention is focused on looking for early responders in early phase and proof-of-principle trials. This is particularly true for renal cancer. This chapter presents a snapshot of the variety of approaches in this pipeline between successful model systems to matured disease-specific phase III trial. The acceptance of new therapy must be anticipated to be contingent on phase III trial testing; to this point, tempered enthusiasm for single-arm trials' results remains appropriate.

The renal cancer population is relatively heterogeneous whether evaluated by conventional histology, prognostic models, site of metastasis, or novel markers. This leads to difficulty in selecting promising approaches based on isolated responders in early-phase trials. Through most of the period of testing, many of the compounds are available for clinical use only in investigational trials. Often the trials have entrance criteria that appear restricted to a fraction of the available, interested population. A common pattern in 2005 is zero or one previous immunotherapy treatment, and clear cell subtype only, and no central nervous system (CNS) metastasis history. For the individual patient seeking a particular compound, a working knowledge of trial databases such as cancer.gov, www.nkca.org, and regional cancer centers may be especially useful. A Web site that incorporates critiques of ongoing trials as well as patient-directed conceptual discussions is cancerguide.org.

Many approaches are in contemporary development (Fig. 8.1). The major categories considered here include drugs that attack conventional targets, that is, DNA or microtubules; "targeted drugs" that affect enzymatic function of other surface, nuclear, or cytoplasmic proteins; drugs influencing general immunity; immune products derived from tumor material; immune maneuvers using leukocytes including T cells, dendritic cells, or stem cells; and finally, treatments attacking the unique physiology of tumor-associated blood vessels. Some therapeutic strategies encompass multiple categories, as do some combination approaches. Any novel approach is potentially of scientific or clinical interest; it is often unclear what "drug class" should be assigned to particular product. New testing approaches and understanding patterns of failure can lead indirectly to improvements of clinical utility.

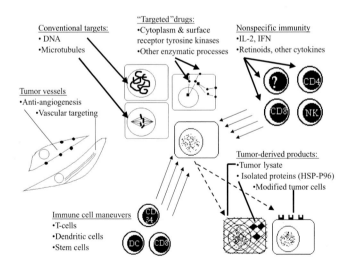

Fig. 8.1. Diagram illustrating the diverse concepts in preclinical and translational application to the problem of therapy for kidney cancer.

Conventional Cytotoxics

Conventional cytotoxic drugs are familiar to the practicing medical oncologist as a class effective for inducing response or cure for many histological categories, but for which renal cancer is the nonresponsive outlier. Although this reputation is generally deserved (see, for example, the table of negative single-arm studies compiled by Amato [1] and more recent citations [2]), there may be several exceptions. Among antimetabolite drugs, trials have demonstrated responses with 5-fluorouracil (5-FU), and the related oral prodrug of that compound, capecitabine. A group of trials developed at University of Chicago used a combination of 21-day continuous infusion 5-FU with 30-minute gemcitabine doses, once a week, on a 28-day cycle with 1 week of no drug. The two-part combination showed response rate of 7 of 41, with additional stable disease in 5 of 41 [3]. Extensions of the regimen, with interleukin-2 (IL-2) and interferon [4], thalidomide [5], and cisplatin [6] showed isolated responses, but did not suggest superiority. Identification of whether there is DNA damage, RNA damage, or interference with another pathway is a consideration for the important mechanism to assign to this nucleoside analogue.

The oral drug capecitabine is converted to 5-FU in a three-enzyme pathway (carboxylesterase, cytidine deaminase, thymidine phosphorylase [TP]), the last of which is potentially concentrated in tumor cells, yielding a theoretically better therapeutic ratio than the parental drug, as well as the more convenient oral route of administration. Gemcitabine has also been combined with capecitabine with 20% response observed at a preliminary report [7]; a similar regimen has been tested in Cancer and Leukemia Group B (CALGB) trial 90008, with 15% (confidence interval [CI] 7–27%) frequency or partial response [8]. These experiences may define a stable point for building a chemotherapy-based approach to renal cancer.

As for single-agent capecitabine and capecitabine in combination with interferon, Wenzel and colleagues [9] in Austria reported that of 23 patients, two had a major response, five had a minor response, and 13 had stable disease, so that a total of 87% of patients had at least stable disease. A U.S. series had a lower response rate, with only 32% stable disease, a result that may have been attributable to selection of a heavily pretreated, refractory population [10]. A newer series from Austria shows a high frequency of stable disease when capecitabine was combined with low-dose IL-2 (4.5 mIU) or with interferon-α (6 mIU three times a week) [11]. This series also showed several patients with major response (5/52), minor response (5/52), and again a high frequency of stable disease (32/52).

Although platinum-containing drugs are among the conventional cytotoxic identified to have low activity in renal cancer (see citations [1]), theoretical synergism with gemcitabine was the basis for a trial using this gemcitabine plus cisplatin combination in kidney cancer (cancer.gov). Combinations with targeted drugs and conventional cytotoxic compounds will test if these classes can be complementary.

Gemcitabine is also part of a two-drug combination with doxorubicin that is to be tested in a single-arm phase II study in sarcomatoid renal cancer. The Eastern Cooperative Oncology Group (ECOG) study will focus on a subtype routinely identified as refractory to medical therapy and as a prognostically unfavorable outlier, even within the general renal cancer group [12].

The novel antimetabolite troxacitabine was tested in a National Cancer Institute (NCI)–Canada phase II study for renal cancer; of 33 patients, two were major responders, and 21 had stable disease, eight of whom were for over 6 months. The mechanism of action of troxacitabine, a stereochemically nonnatural nucleoside analogue, is chain termination, interfering with the function of mammalian DNA polymerases [13]. Additional testing with this compound may yield a more favorable way to extend the duration of stable disease, or increase the frequency of major responses.

Among drugs directed at the microtubule, vinblastine is notable for having been the single agent on the inferior arm of the most favorable randomized phase III trial of interferon plus vinblastine versus vinblastine [14]. A similarly pessimistic conclusion was reached in single-arm trials of the taxane docetaxel [15–17]. The epothilone compounds are derived from a soil bacterium, *Sorangium cellulosum*, instead of plant parent compounds. The site of contact with tubulin is the same as that of taxanes, and point mutations (not identified to be common in kidney cancer) inhibit responsiveness to either drug [18]. However, non–cross-resistance has been observed in some early testing. The difference may be related to drug efflux or to a nonmicrotubule target. Patupilone (EP0906, Novartis East Hanover, NJ) and Ixabepilone (BMS247550, Bristol-Myers Squib, Princeton,

NJ). The latter is the treatment plan in a single-arm phase II renal cell cancer (RCC) trial at the NCI, and 10% partial responses in kidney cancer were reported in June 2004 [19]. Additional microtubule targeting drugs are discussed below (see "Vascular Targeting").

Key determinants of renal cancer resistance to conventional cytotoxic drugs remain to be identified and circumvented. Teleologically, the kidney is an organ that must resist and expel toxic substances, and this may be part of the basis for the recalcitrance of renal cancer to conventional cytotoxic treatment. Drugs directed at the adenosine triphosphate (ATP)-binding cassette (ABC) transporter drugs, such as P-glycoprotein (Pgp), multidrug resistance–related protein (MRP), and breast cancer resistance protein (BCRP) are another category of compounds that may ultimately have relevance for improving the outcomes for conventional cytotoxic drugs in renal cancer.

Targeted Drugs

Targeted drug therapy has become the watchword of the pharmaceutical industry in the new millennium. Isolated successes such as rituximab for non-Hodgkin lymphoma or imatinib mesylate in chronic myelogenous leukemia are a basis for hope that each cancer will have a pharmacogenomically discoverable Achilles' heel, susceptible to the right target/targeted drug combination, with inconsequential toxicity. The targets of renal cancer remain elusive. Pathophysiological studies highlight the pathway related to von Hippel–Lindau protein (pVHL), mutated or silent in over half of cases [20]. Within this pathway, the impaired degradation of the hypoxia-inducible factor 1α (HIF1α) protein and the consequent dysregulated (increased) transcription of genes bearing the hypoxia response element (HRE) sequence in their promoter are leading candidates to be a major contributor to the pathological phenotype of clear cell renal cancer. The dysregulated activity of HIF1α- and HRE-bearing genes is found in other kidney cancer and many other malignancies. Many investigational approaches in preclinical testing that target HIF directly include, small interfering siRNA and others, such as small molecules and novel agents already in clinical testing [21,22]. Vascular endothelial growth factor (VEGF) is a gene product with HRE regulation. VEGF-depleting drugs and

VEGF receptor (VEGFR1 or Flt-1 and VEGFR2 or Flk-1/KDR) in tyrosine kinase enzyme inhibitors are discussed below (see "Angiogenic Targeting"), although the pathology caused by VEGF likely extends beyond the recruitment of blood vessel growth and lymphatic vessel growth into the tumor and may include immune impairment or direct tumor stimulation.

Receptor tyrosine kinase inhibitors and antibodies or other drugs that block the external domains of these receptors are in broad development in oncology. The epidermal growth factor receptor (EGFR) is targeted by small molecule drugs gefitinib (ZD1839, Iressa™), erlotinib (Tarceva™), and CI-1033 (also blocks Her2/neu, EGFR3, and EGFR4 tyrosine kinases), and by antibodies such as cetuximab (Erbitux™, Bristol-Myers Squib, C225). Diverse trials of gefitinib monotherapy and in combination with cytotoxic drugs have led to its approval for non–small-cell lung cancer. Two single-agent gefitinib trials in renal cancer have been reported; one trial of 16 patients demonstrated a response in none, with only three patients not progressing at 4 months [23], and the other trial of 21 patients reported a major response in none and stable disease in eight (38%) [24]. The SD patients had significantly better survival [24]. Although these gefitinib trials suggest that chronic oral EGFR tyrosine kinase inhibition is a blockade and is not relevant in renal cancer, the chemically related drug erlotinib (Tarceva™) is in active trials as well. Two of these are a second-line therapy of renal cancer (NCI Web site), and essentially the only phase II trial directed exclusively at therapy of the papillary histology subset (Southwest Oncology Group [SWOG] trial 0317). Another trial testing the combination of erlotinib and the anti-VEGF antibody bevacizumab was presented positively at the June 2004 American Society of Clinical Oncology (ASCO) meeting and recently published [25]. Among 59 evaluable patients reported, 15 (25%) had partial response and 36 (61%) had stable disease or minor response at 8 weeks, with median progression free survival of 11 months, and 60% survival at 18 months. Rash, diarrhea, and nausea were the most frequent side effects. A randomized trial of bevacizumab with or without erlotinib has completed accrual.

The small molecule inhibitor sunitinib malate (also called Su11248, Su011248, brand name Sutent™, Pfizer, New York, NY) is an orally available tyrosine kinase inhibitor of VEGFR2, PDGFR, flt3, and c-*kit*. A phase III study with randomization versus interferon has completed accrual. Favorable data were presented at the June 2004 ASCO meeting and have now been published. The published report describes 63 evaluable patients who had progressed after prior treatment with a single line of immunotherapy; 25 of them (40%) had a partial response (PR), and 17 more (27%) had stable disease at least 3 months, and the median time to progression was reached at 8.7 months [26]. The drug was approved in January 2006 by the U.S. FDA, based on the experience in this trial and a second, similar single arm trial.

The proteasome inhibitor bortezimib has also been tested for renal cancer. The proteasome is the site of degradation of ubiquitylated proteins, many of which are involved in the cell cycle. Proteasome inhibition may have impact on HIF1α levels. In one single-agent phase II series, there was one objective response in 21 patients [27]. In an independent series, there were three responses among 24 clear cell subtype patients, which may be encouraging for exploring further development of this unique class of agents [28].

The drug CCI-779 (Wyeth) is an inhibitor of the mammalian target of rapamycin (mTOR) protein. Several intracellular signaling processes function through mTOR, which interacts with HIF1a, the PI3K/Akt pathway, and cell cycle proteins including cyclin D1 (leading to a late-G1 arrest from mTOR inhibition). This point of cytoplasmic interference is not just a new target protein but a new point of attack in the growth and survival of the malignant cell cycle. A randomized phase II study in renal cancer, using dose levels of 25 mg/m^2, 75 mg/m^2, or 250 mg/m^2 was reported by Atkins et al. [29]. There were no differences identified across dose levels, and the 25 mg/m^2 dose has been selected for further study in renal cancer. Among 111 patients, the observed response rate was 7%, with an additional 26% minor responses. Most frequent toxicities were rash and mucositis. The median time to progression and overall survival were 5.8 months and 15 months, respectively. The prognostic criteria of Motzer et al. [30] identified intermediate and poor subsets, which appeared to have a better improvement of progression-free survival. Atkins et al. [29] speculate that a relationship to the Akt pathway in these patients may be basis for this observation. A randomized phase III study of CCI-779, interferon, and CCI-779 plus interferon is open at international centers, restricted to worse-prognosis patients [30]. A single-arm phase I study of CCI-779 plus interferon in renal cancer has also been presented [31].

Finally, an exciting development in 2003 that was reported at the ASCO 2004 meeting was the single-agent phase II study of sorafenib (brand name Nexavar™, previously called Bay 43-9006) [32]. The small-molecule inhibits (at different levels) b-*raf*, c-*raf*, PDGFRβ, c-*kit*, *flt*-3, and VEGF-R2 (KDR). The Raf proteins are involved in signal transduction from cell surface receptor molecules, in the widely present RAS/RAF/MEK/MAPK pathway [33].

The Bay43-9006 study design originally emphasized colon cancer until it was evident that RCC appears as the most responsive of the histological types tested. The design has a three-part plan at the 12-week evaluation: subjects with 25% improvement are continued on treatment, those with >25% worsening are discontinued for progression, and those with stable disease are offered randomization between placebo and continued treatment. Among the 45 patients meeting the rule for randomization, a significant prolonged time to progression was observed for those assigned to a second 12 weeks of drug than to placebo. In the pivotal randomized, double blind placebo controlled phase III trial comparing sorafenib to placebo, time to progression was improved with (24 weeks versus 12 weeks, $p < .000001$ [34]. Seventy-four percent (versus 20% on placebo) had some tumor shrinkage, but the "partial response" frequency was lower than in the sunitinib phase II trial of A planned intermediate survival analysis (220 events, with final analysis planned at 540 events) showed hazard ratio of 0.72 (which did not meet the planned early evaluation statistical significance of .00005) is encouraging that the trial may also demonstrate a median survival benefit [34]. The eventual survival comparison will be "contaminated" by crossover from the placebo to the active treatment when the trial was unblinded based on the progression free survival data. Side effects of hypertension, rash, and hand–foot syndrome were observed, but were predominantly low grade. Sunitinib and sorafenib, representing the first major kidney cancer drug approvals in over a decade, will have a wide impact on the treatment of kidney cancer. The best way to bring the targeted drug paradigm to bear for longer, complete responses in renal cancer is a task for subsequent empiric experience, in the hopeful context of several active non–cross-resistant drugs. Combination with other drugs affecting cell surface receptor tyrosine kinase, RAS/RAF/MEK/MAP pathway, and common points such as the proteasome or mTOR can be anticipated to be of interest in renal and other cancers. Complex interactions, such as VEGFR-mediated resistance to EGFR blockade [25] may be important and only revealed in combination applications, several of which are in trials described at cancer.gov.

General Immunity

Although sometimes stereotyped as "the chemotherapy nonresponder," kidney cancer, particularly the clear cell subtype, is also considered to be "immune-sensitive." Partly on this basis, and notwithstanding that many cancer types are immune-sensitive in murine models, it is kidney cancer that is a frequent focus of the translational effort of immunotherapy. Some of these novel treatments build on IL-2 or interferon therapy. Specific immunity vaccine approaches are discussed in the next section. The mechanisms of immune evasion by renal cancers, and by cancers in general, are undoubtedly complex. Some of the cytokines elaborated by tumors are known to have anergy-favoring effects on the immune systems, including transforming growth factor-β (TGF-β), IL-10, and VEGF. The ultimate therapeutic attack may involve directly negating this effect, or circumventing it through a different immune-enhancing maneuver.

The cytokine IL-12 influences dendritic cell function, favoring promotion of cellular immunity, including possibly useful antitumor immunity. Striking synergy of IL-12 plus IL-2 in murine models [35] has been encouraging. Practical synergy is yet to be demonstrated. A phase I trial using six doses of high-dose bolus IL-2, given in groups of three with IL-12 on intervening days, is open at NCI, and a phase I trial using IL-12 with interferon has been reported [36]. Hematological and hepatic toxicity were observed. Two of 18 kidney cancer patients in the trial had responses, a preliminary efficacy assessment.

Antibody drugs that suppress the CTLA4+ (CD152) cell subset (corresponding to the suppressors lymphocytes, also identified as Treg) had good success in some murine tumor models [37,38], and an immunologically detectable effect in vaccinated cancer patients [39]. A phase II single-arm study of MDX 010 (Medarex, Princeton, NY), for IL-2 refractory or ineligible patients is open at the National Institutes of Health (NIH). The optimal use of this type of manipulation of the immune system will undoubtedly be in combination with other available immune maneuvers and treatments. One may anticipate that combination development will be contingent on the single-agent experience.

Thalidomide is a drug with many proposed mechanisms of action. The relevant mechanism of action is unknown, but may be immune modulation or downregulation of cytokines, including tumor necrosis factor-α (TNF-α), VEGF, basic fibroblast growth factor (bFGF), or IL-12, as well as interfering with some step of angiogenesis. The antiangiogenic and immune-modulation mechanisms were the key rationales for application testing in several series of RCC clinical trials. The dominant response reported was disease stabilization, although some series identified some partial responders [40–44]. A safe conclusion across these series appears to be that at best the impact of the drug is on a minority of patients, the observed disease stabilization is not of conclusive survival benefit, and further single-agent testing is unlikely to show an impact on median survival.

Disparate results were identified in two single-arm trials combining the drug with IL-2. Amato et al. [45] reported a major response frequency of 39% (two complete responses [CR] and 11 PR among 37 evaluable patients) using a regimen of 4 weeks of 5-day-a-week IL-2 at 7 million IU/m^2 plus thalidomide 200 mg/d. Additionally, 10 patients had stable disease. Formal publication is awaited; a trial using the same two agents with the addition of granulocyte-macrophage colony-stimulating factor (GM-CSF) as an antigen presentation enhancing drug has been opened [46]. In contrast, Olencki et al. [47] found three responders in 33 patients with a regimen of thalidomide 100 mg/d and IL-2 at 250,000 IU/kg during week 1 and 125,000 IU/kg during weeks 2 to 6. Two related drugs, CC4017 (Actimid^{TM}) and CC5013, (Revlimid^{TM} and lenolidomide Celgene, Summit, NJ) have potent in vitro effects on lymphocytes as well as on TNF-α. These newer analogues appear to lack the teratogenicity risk and neuropathy problem that have been pervasive in efforts to expand the oncological application of thalidomide. One may anticipate the potential for testing in kidney cancer; a single-agent phase II renal cancer study with lenolidomide is open at Baylor University [48] and other centers.

A cooperative group phase III randomized trial of low-dose interferon-α2b (3 million units three times a week vs. interferon plus thalidomide) has been presented (E2898). It addressed the issue of whether the thalidomide plus interferon combination is active in renal cancer, by antiangiogenesis or another mechanism. The results presented in June 2004 revealed an extremely low response in the control arm (2.2%), and a response of 6.5% in the combination arm. There were more thrombotic events (12 vs. 4)

in the combination arm, the median progression-free survival favored the combination (2.8 vs. 3.8 months, $p = .04$), and the overall survival favored (nonsignificantly) the control arm (12.2 vs. 10.8 months) [49].

Finally, pharmacokinetic modifications of IL-2 and interferon have been developed. The Bayer compound BAY 50-4798 is an analogue of natural IL-2, but with modification to activate T cells but not natural killer (NK) cells. This may have a favorable effect on toxicity. Considering that the relevant mechanism of action of IL-2 remains a subject of controversy—one view is that for renal cancer it is the NK cells that are more relevant than CD8+ T cells (as may be the case in melanoma)—further disease-specific clinical testing will certainly be warranted. Subcutaneous pegylated interferons have a longer half-life and a higher molecular weight compared to unmodified interferon (molecular weight 19,000 to 20,000 dalton). Available pegylated interferons, with indications for treatment of infectious hepatitis, used in combination with Ribavirin include Pegasys™ (interferon-α2a, molecular weight 60,000, manufactured by Roche, Basel, Switzerland) and Pegintron™ (interferon-α2b, molecular weight 31,000, manufactured by Schering-Plough, Kenilworth, NJ) [50,51]. Anticancer testing of interferon-α2a for renal cancer showed five PR (19%) among 27 patients treated in the phase I testing, [52]; the recommended dose for further testing was 450 mg once a week. There was one CR and four PRs (overall 13%) among 40 previously untreated renal cancer patients in the phase II experience [53]. The report of phase I to II testing of the trial of pegylated interferon-α2b in renal cancer determined a dose of 6 mg/kg/week, with the observation that some patients could tolerate 7.5 mg/kg/week. Thirty-five previously untreated renal cell cancer patients were in the phase II part of the trial; 23 of 57 had at least stable disease at week 12. Objective response was observed in 6 of the 44 evaluable previously untreated renal cancer patients. At 1 year, two CRs and four PRs (overall 11% of the 57) were ongoing [54], and a total of 44 previously untreated renal cell cancer patients were evaluable for response.

Leukocyte Products

In the preclinical experience, nucleated blood cells have enormous potential for therapeutic immune manipulation. Ex vivo isolation, sorting, expansion, and activation seem to define an untenable

matrix of testable approaches. Historically tested methods, including tumor infiltrating lymphocytes (TIL) [55,56] and autologous lymphocyte infusion (ALT) [55], offer ready contexts for new variations, such as cell sorting and ex vivo cytokine application. The open single-arm trial in St. Luke's Medical Center (Milwaukee, WI) uses IL-2 and anti-CD3 activating antibodies on the apheresis-derived lymphocytes, which are reinfused to subjects [58].

A special case of leukocyte-derived novel therapies involve use of dendritic cells (DCs), the major antigen-presenting cell type. Monocyte-derived DCs may be prepared from the apheresis product by culture of adherent mononuclear cells, which are then exposed to GM-CSF and IL-4. These autologous, human leukocyte antigen (HLA)-matched DCs may then be loaded with antigen in a variety of ways, and then reintroduced.

Vieweg's group [59] has explored the use of nucleic acid material to load DCs. The messenger RNA (mRNA) of tumor cells may encompass tumor-specific antigens, with advantages over protein-based approaches in that it may be nonspecifically amplified as needed using standard techniques. Similarly, RNA coding for selected antigens, such as telomerase protein (TERT), present in the whole-tumor derived mRNA, can be used to load DCs, offering both the advantage of emphasizing specific tumor antigens, as well as a specific strategy for monitoring response to a single protein. The acquisition of cytotoxic T lymphocyte (CTL) with this specificity was identified with the acquisition of polyclonal CTL, in six of seven evaluated patients in a 10-patient clinical trial. The clinical implication of the immune changes remain uncertain, as most subjects took other therapy after the study treatment.

Dendritic cells physiologically take up apoptotic bodies. Another vaccine approach, recently reported in non–small-cell lung cancer patients, is with allogeneic tumor cells, treated with ultraviolet (UV) radiation to induce apoptosis and admixed with autologous DCs. Acquisition of T cells with antitumor specificity was detectable by, enzyme linked immunospot (ELISPOT) assay [60]. The ex vivo fusion of dendritic cells with autologous tumor cells is a way to introduce cells bearing both the in situ particular antigen and the HLA repertoire of the tumor and competent antigen-presentation cell surface molecules. Avigan and colleagues [61] described a clinical trial applying this technique. Among 13 renal cancer patients treated, five had disease

stabilization for 3 to 9 months; two breast cancer patients had responses, one durable for more than 24 months. Practical drawbacks include the need for three separate ex vivo cellular manipulations: single-cell suspension of autologous tumor, apheresis of peripheral blood mononuclear cells for DC culture, and cell fusion with verification of presence of biphenotypic (tumor and DC) cells for vaccine administration. In the cited report, 32 subjects had successful product preparation, and 23 of 58 enrolled subjects were actually treated, with products having 28% to 71% fusion efficiency.

A groundbreaking investigational clear cell renal cancer therapy is based on transfer of stem cells is the nonmyeloablative allogeneic stem cell transplant. The seminal publication in 2000 showed 9 of 19 patients (who had disease refractory to IL-2) demonstrating at least partial responses, attributable to the graft versus tumor (GVT) effect. Three had complete responses [62]. Additional experience including from Europe and from other centers will be critical in defining the best patient selection criteria and graft-versus-host management [63,64].

In the nonmyeloablative transplant technique, the path to the therapeutic outcome can be considered as separate steps. The first is selection of a suitable patient and suitable donor. In the initial experience at NCI, favorable responses were seen essentially only in the clear cell subtype, and the worldwide experience emphasizes this subtype. (Treatment of individuals with a histological type that is not clear cell, an even more heterogeneous group, remains an area for exploration, as the current series emphasize or require the clear cell type.)

Because the time until therapeutic effect may be long, a further requirement is that the patient will be able to survive until the therapeutic effect becomes apparent. The ideal donor is most frequently defined as an HLA-identical (nonidentical twin) full sibling, who is an individual with mismatches of other alleles (minor antigens). Alternative donors, such as partial mismatch siblings or matched unrelated donors, are another area in active exploration, because it appears that the frequency of patients who have donors meeting the first criterion is limited; for example, only 84 of 284 (29.6%) at University of Chicago had donors that could be screened [65]. Besides the limitations on donors, limitations on histological subtype, rate of growth of the tumor, sites of tumor, and comorbidities can be anticipated to continue to limit applicability of the method.

A next step is manipulation of the graft material obtained by apheresis. For example, this can include depletion of lymphocytes to a defined dose. Preparative chemotherapy for the host is directed at host lymphocytes, and of lower intensity than in a traditional myeloablative stem cell transplant, such as for a hematological malignancy. Fludarabine and cyclophosphamide combinations have been used, with an emphasis on marrow ablation, not antitumor effect. After graft infusion, the extent of engraftment may be monitored. Complete donor chimerism may be a necessary intermediate goal. Subsequently, discontinuation of immune suppression, as well as donor lymphocyte infusions (DLIs) to support the graft, can be used, titrated against observed graft-versus-host disease. General immune-function deficits may require antibacterial, antiviral, and antifungal support. Finally, hands-on management of graft-versus-host disease, with a variety of immune suppressive drugs including steroids, cyclosporine, methotrexate, and others, is requisite.

Tumor Products

Cellular material for therapeutic use can also be obtained directly from the tumor. As mentioned above, tumor material can be used to obtain peptide, nucleic acid, or other material for loading into dendritic cells. Tumor cell material may also be used without ex vivo dendritic cell loading. Presumably antigen presentation can occur in vivo with either the modified tumor cell acting as substitute antigen-presenting cell, or attracting autologous dendritic cells that then take up the relevant antigen and process and present it effectively.

The Oncophage™ product, in phase III RCC testing, uses heat shock protein and the associated peptides obtained from fresh tumor (HSPPC-96) as the material for the loading of DCs. This set of peptides has the feature that it contains peptides that will be loaded onto cell surface major histocompatibility complex (MHC) molecules, and so may represent an immunogenically useful panel to which to stimulate a response. The mixture may be particularly well acquired for processing by dendritic cells [66,67]. Some published studies indicate that this strategy is sufficient to induce measurable, apparently useful antitumor immunity, even in the context of a cancer that had been metastatic [68]. Two randomized studies using Oncophage seek to enroll either patients having nephrectomy in the face of metastatic disease or patients having nephrectomy for cure, but for whom tumor, node, metastasis (TNM) staging is consistent with a high recurrence risk [69].

Our group has worked with B7.1 transduced autologous tumor cell vaccine that is irradiated and then given sequentially before an outpatient schedule of subcutaneous IL-2. Upon resection of tumor material, often primary tumor but also metastasis, short-term tissue culture is used and then the dendritic cell surface co-stimulatory protein B7.1 is introduced with a viral vector. Theoretically this would allow naive lymphocytes with antitumor specificity to encounter tumor antigens in the context of this "second signal" (B7.1 on the antigen-presenting cell, CD28 on the lymphocyte) that would promote activation over anergy or deletion [70]. A different cytokine that tumor cells can be modified to release is GM-CSF. This localized secretion of GM-CSF should recruit dendritic cells that will process the antigen [71]. The GVAX® products (cell Genesys, South San Francisco, CA) are in trial in several cancer subtypes, uses this strategy [72].

The autologous tumor lysate (aTL) product was the subject of a randomized phase III adjuvant trial in Germany for which progression-free survival results were reported in 2004. For this vaccine, the tumor cells are in culture for several hours in media containing interferon-γ and tocopherol, and then devitalized with freeze/thaw cycling. The former should induce higher expression of MHC cell surface molecules, causing an enhanced immunogenicity. The reported results—the only large, randomized vaccine renal cancer trial conducted in Europe—are consistent with an improvement in time-to-detected progression [73]. An apparent imbalance of the attrition in patients randomized to active treatment, and the unreported overall survival data, among other factors, may limit interpretation of the clinical outcome data [74].

In common across all of these tumor cell–derived therapeutic products is a product safety infrastructure. This includes the need for product characterization, irradiation of potentially live tumor cell material, monitoring for bacterial or other contaminants, and explicit vaccine material/patient matching. The decision about which aspects of the product must be monitored may be a difficult one. A continued reference to the huge theoretical potency of specific anticancer immunotherapy is required to justify this significant infrastructure and expense.

Angiogenic Targeting

Renal cancer specimens are often observed to be densely vascu-
larized; reports of difficult-to-control bleeding during surgery on
metastases (as opposed to nephrectomy, where the renal vascular
stalk is a point of control) are common. The concept of targeting
the blood vessels of the cancer is appealing for several reasons:
low toxicity, conversion of the disease to a chronic pattern, and
an independent attack at a fundamental vulnerability of the
growing tumor. The genotype of the targeted cell type is theoretically stable and comparable across cancer subtypes. A variety of
drugs have been validated as members of the antiangiogenic
class, using in vitro and murine models. The transition to clinical application has been slow, but includes some testing in kidney
cancer, in addition to renal cancer patients who have participated
in phase studies. In contrast to conventional cytotoxic drugs, an
emphasis could be on nontoxic disease stabilization rather than
on regression. Thalidomide and related compounds and Su11248
are discussed above [75,76].

Vascular endothelial growth factor A (VEGF-A), which is
present in several isoforms [77], is the ligand of cell surface receptors [VEGF-R1 (*flt-1*), VEGF-R2 (*flk*), and VEGF-R3]. The VEGF
levels may be high in RCC, relating to HRE in the gene promoter.
Other VEGF gene family members (VEGF-B, VEGF-C, VEGF-D,
VEGF-E) may have other diverse roles in cancer [78]. Presence of
receptors on tumor blood vessels identifies blocking of the
VEGF/VEGFR pathway as an appealing target. Depletion of free
VEGF occurs with bevacizumab (Avastin™, Genentech, South San
Francisco, CA), a 93% humanized antibody, approved for colorectal cancer [79]. The VEGF-TRAP drug, a synthetic protein
composed of domains of the immunoglobulin Fc, and extra-
cellular domains of *flt-1* and *flk*, appears to have the same general
mechanism of action [80].

In a randomized phase II trial of bevacizumab for progressive,
refractory renal cancer, a high frequency of stable disease was
identified in the high-dose arm (64% at 4 months, vs. 20% for the
placebo group). Major responses were observed in four of 40
patients (10%), and multiyear stabilizations were identified as
well [81]. Clinical testing of combinations with interferon and IL-
2, are in trials as the optimal use of bevacizumab for renal cancer
is developed. A cooperative group CALGB trial of interferon with
or without bevacizumab is open [82]. Side effects observed in the

experience to this point include risk of bleeding and hypertension. The bevacizumab plus erlotinib trial is cited above.

Vascular Targeting

Vascular targeting drugs employ a different strategy. A transient direct attack on the tumor endothelium may result in tumor infarction. Combretastatin is one member of this group that targets endothelial cell microtubules, for which phase I trials have been completed [83,84]. Measurement of tumor blood flow, for example by dynamic contrast magnetic resonance imaging (DC-MRI), may provide a method to identify the occurrence of vascular blockade by this class of drugs. Another member of the class for which phase I testing was completed is ZD6126 (AstraZeneca, Wilmington, DE), and ABT-751 (Abbott, Chicago, IL), which is orally available, was tested in a phase II company-sponsored renal cancer trial. A review of many of these agents suggests that one may anticipate their development for renal cancer [85]. The vascular targeting drugs remain in an early stage of development.

A natural product drug, Neovastat (AE-941, Aeterna Laboratories, Quebec city, Quebec, Canada) may affect VEGF-related signaling and inhibit matrix metalloproteases. For classification purposes, the mechanism of action for this cartilage-derived substance can be considered as a multifunctional antiangiogenesis. A favorable subset analysis from a multidiagnosis trial that had 22 evaluable renal cancer patients suggested that a higher dose was consistent with a survival benefit [86,87]. A randomized phase III kidney cancer trial has completed accrual and was negative, but again a subject for which favorable outcome from the drug was identified.

Conclusion

The process of developing a concept, translational testing, verification of targets, and clinical trials takes years. The complex intracellular and immunological targets and numerous classes of drugs seem to define an unending array of testable strategies. Development strategies depend both on conceptual priorities and on practical (economic) realization issues of pharmaceutical companies. Renal cancer, therefore, is often not the initial development target, and a significant amount of experience in other histologies with a particular strategy may accrue before any formal testing is done in renal cancer. Conversely, early responses observed in renal cancer have been met with enthusiastic, significant trial infrastructure investment, including for CCI-779, sorafenib, bevacizumab, and sunitinib. Besides biological theory, there will be the relevance of this other experience, obviously more appealing in the case of positive trials, weighing on the decision process.

For patients seeking treatment in 2006, the role of sorafenib and sunitinib is evolving. The novelty and ability to titrate the oral medicines are appealing. Limitations of the off-study therapies may put investigational vaccines, compounds, and combinations in the forefront. A practical approach is to canvas available treatments, using Web sites and personal contacts, and to then try to reach a rapid decision. Despite an understandable ambition to get a chance at access to every promising drug, the therapeutic plan must integrate logistic issues and the uncertain appeal of theoretical mechanisms of action. Patients, even those with slowly progressing disease, may have relatively limited realistic options for participation in clinical trials.

Among key compounds in later phase trials in 2006 include sorafenib, sunitinib, CCI-779, and bevacizumab. Some immune manipulations are similarly centered on single drugs, such as the MDX-010 antibody or IL-12. Older drugs, such as high-dose IL-2 (still the only regimen with occasional long-term disease-free survivors), IL-2 and interferon combinations, and phase I drugs, are typically part of the discussion as well.

Many immune manipulations are more complex, such as non-myeloablative transplant or combinations of vaccines or immune modulators with IL-2 or interferon. Trials frequently focus on never-treated or once-treated/now-progressing subsets. Conversely, the prevalent patient population interested in new therapy is a group more heterogeneous for comorbidities, extent of pretreatment, and distribution of metastatic disease, especially brain metastasis.

From where will the next breakthrough treatment for renal cancer come? What will be the best use of sorafenib and sunitinib? Of targeted-immunotherapy combinations? Notwithstanding the uncertainty of enthusiasm derived from single-arm trials, the targeted drugs appear to be a frontrunner category. Each additional drug with an indication for renal cancer will almost certainly have a toxicity profile better than cytokine (IL-2, interferon) approaches and may change the face of therapeutic planning for metastatic RCC. One may remain hopeful that the paradigm shift toward targeted, tolerated, durable metastatic RCC management can emerge from the many contemporary approaches to the problem.

Controversies and Outstanding Issues

1. Is there any role for any adjuvant therapy?
2. Are there biological markers for response to individual agents?
3. Are these agents to be used as monotherapy or in combination?

References

1. Amato RJ. Chemotherapy for renal cell carcinoma. Semin Oncol 2000;27(2):177–16.
2. Fishman M, Antonia S. Novel therapies for renal cell carcinoma—an update. Expert Opin Investig Drugs 2003;12(4):593–609.
3. Rini BL, Vogezang NJ, Dumas MC, Wade JL, Taber DA, Stadlet WM. Phase II trial of weekly intravenous gemcitabine with continuous infusion fluorouracil in patients with metastatic renal cell cancer. J Clin Oncol 2000;18(12):2419–2426.
4. Ryan CW, Vogezang NJ, Stadler WM. A phase II trial of intravenous gemcitabine and 5–fluorouracil with subcutaneous interleukin-2 and interferon-alpha in patients with metastatic renal cell carcinoma. Cancer 2002;94(10):2602–2609.
5. Desai AA, Vogezang NJ, Rini B, et al. A phase II trial of weekly intravenous gemcitabine (G) with prolonged continuous infusion 5–fluorouracil (F) and oral thalidomide (T) in patients with metastatic renal cell cancer (mRCC). Proc Am Soc Clin Oncol 2001;(abstr 2448).
6. George CM, Vogezang NJ, Rini BI, et al. A phase II trial of weekly intravenous gemcitabine and cisplatin with continuous infusion fluorouracil in patients with metastatic renal cell carcinoma. Ann Oncol 2002;13(1):116–120.
7. Waters JS, Moss C, Hackett S, et al. A phase II trial of gemcitabine (GEM) plus capecitabine (CAPE) in patients with metastatic renal cell carcinoma (MRCC). Proc Am Soc Clin Oncol 2003;22:386(abstr 1549).

8. Stadler WM, Halabi S, Ernstoff MS, et al. A phase II study of gemcitabine (G) and capecitabine (C) in patients with metastatic renal cell cancer (mRCC): a report of Cancer and Leukemia Group B #90008. Proc Am Soc Clin Oncol 2004;23:(abstr 4515).

9. Wenzel C, Locker GJ, Bartsch R, et al. Capecitabine monotherapy and in combination with immunotherapy in the treatment of metastatic renal cell carcinoma. Anticancer Drugs 2003;14(10):779–784.

10. Chang DZ, Olencki T, Budd GT, et al. Phase I trial of capecitabine in combination with interferon alpha in patients with metastatic renal cancer: toxicity and pharmacokinetics. Cancer Chemother Pharmacol 2001;48(6):493–498.

11. Wenzel C, Locker GJ, Schmidinger M, et al. Capecitabine in the treatment of metastatic renal cell carcinoma failing immunotherapy. Am J Kidney Dis 2002;39(1):48–54.

12. Cheville JC, Lohse CM, Zincke H, et al. Sarcomatoid renal cell carcinoma: an examination of underlying histologic subtype and an analysis of associations with patient outcome. Am J Surg Pathol 2004;28(4):435–441.

13. Townsley CA, Chi K, Ernst DS, et al. Phase II study of troxacitabine (BCH-4556) in patients with advanced and/or metastatic renal cell carcinoma: a trial of the National Cancer Institute of Canada-Clinical Trials Group. J Clin Oncol 2003;21(8):1524–1529.

14. Pyrhonen S, Salminen E, Ruutu M, et al. Prospective randomized trial of interferon alfa-2a plus vinblastine versus vinblastine alone in patients with advanced renal cell cancer. J Clin Oncol 1999;17:2859–2867.

15. Mertens WC, Eisenhauer EA, Jolivet J, Ernst S, Moore M, Muldal A. Docetaxel in advanced renal carcinoma. A phase II trial of the National Cancer Institute of Canada Clinical Trials Group. Ann Oncol 1994;5(2):185–187.

16. Bruntsch U, Heinrich B, Kaye SB, et al. Docetaxel (Taxotere) in advanced renal cell cancer. A phase II trial of the EORTC Early Clinical Trials Group. Eur J Cancer 1994;30A(8):1064–1067.

17. Sternberg J, Berry M, Gregurich M, Boxer M, Anthony S. Phase-II trial of single-agent, weekly docetaxel in advanced or metastatic renal cell carcinoma (MRCC). Proc Am Soc Clin Oncol 2001;(abstr 2379).

18. Ojima I, Chakravarty S, Inoue T, et al. A common pharmacophore for cytotoxic natural products that stabilize microtubules. Proc Natl Acad Sci USA 1999;96(8):4256–4261.

19. Zhuang SH, Menefee M, Kotz H, et al. A phase II clinical trial of BMS-247550 (ixabepilone), a microtubule-stabilizing agent in renal cell cancer. Proc Am Soc Clin Oncol 2004;(abstr 4550).

20. Brauch H, Weirich G, Brieger J, et al. VHL alterations in human clear cell renal cell carcinoma: association with advanced tumor stage and a novel hot spot mutation. Cancer Res 2000;60(7):1942–1948.

21. Tan C, Roecker AJ, Noronha R, et al. Identification of a small molecule inhibitor of hypoxia-inducible factor (HIF) pathway. American Association for Cancer Research, (AACR) 2004;(abstr 2047).
22. Kline ER, Feng Y, Pribluda V, Lavallee T, Giannakakou P. Translational inhibition of HIF-1α by 2ME2. AACR 2004;(abstr 5428).
23. Drucker B, Bacik J, Ginsberg M, et al. Phase II trial of ZD1839 (IRESSA) in patients with advanced renal cell carcinoma. Invest New Drugs 2003;21(3):341–345.
24. Dawson NA, Guo C, Zak R, et al. A phase II trial of ZD1839 in stage IV and recurrent renal cell carcinoma. Proc Am Soc Clin Oncol 2003;22:404(abstr 1623).
25. Hainsworth JD, Sosman JA, Spigel DR, et al. Treatment of metastatic renal cell carcinoma with a combination of bevacizumab and erlotinib. J Clin Oncol 2005;23:7889–7896.
26. Motzer RJ, Michaelson MD, Redman BG, et al. Activity of SU11248, a multitargeted inhibitor of vascular endothelial growth factor receptor and platelet-derived growth factor receptor, in patients with metastatic renal cell carcinoma. J Clin Oncol 2006;24:16–24.
27. Davis NB, Taber DA, Ansari RH, et al. Phase II trial of PS-341 in patients with renal cell cancer: a University of Chicago Phase II Consortium Study. J Clin Oncol 2004;1:115–119.
28. Drucker BJ, Schwartz L, Bacik J, Mazumdar M, Marion S, Motzer RJ. Phase II trial of PS-341 shows response in patients with advanced renal cell carcinoma. Proc Am Soc Clin Oncol 2003;22:386(abstr 1550).
29. Atkins MB, Hidalgo M, Stadler WM, et al. Randomized phase II study of multiple dose levels of CCI-779, a novel mammalian target of rapamycin kinase inhibitor, in patients with advanced refractory renal cell carcinoma. J Clin Oncol 2004;22(5):909–918.
30. Motzer RJ, Mazumdar M, Bacik J, Berg W, Amsterdam A, Ferrara J. Survival and prog-nostic stratification of 670 patients with advanced renal cell carcinoma. J Clin Oncol 1999;17(8):2530.
31. Smith JW, Ko Y-J, Dutcher J, et al. Update of a phase 1 study of intravenous CCI-779 given in combination with interferon to patients with advanced renal cell carcinoma. Proc Am Soc Clin Oncol 2004;(abstr 385).
32. Ratain MJ, Flaherty KT, Stadler WM, et al. Preliminary antitumor activity of BAY 43–9006 in metastatic renal cell carcinoma and other advanced refractory solid tumors in a phase II randomized discontinuation trial (RDT). Proc Am Soc Clin Oncol 2004;(abstr 382).
33. Beeram M, Patnaik A, Rowinsky EK. Raf: A strategic target for therapeutic development against cancer. J Clin Oncol 2005;23:6771–6790.
34. Escudier B. Randomized phase III trial of the multi-kinase inhibitor sorafenib (BAY 43-9006) in patients with advanced renal cell carcinoma. Abstract # 794. 11/3/2005. ECCO XIII conference (Paris).

35. Wigginton JM, Komschlies KL, Back TC. Administration of inter-leukin 12 with pulse interleukin 2 and the rapid and complete erad-ication of murine renal carcinoma. J Natl Cancer Inst 1996;88:38–43.
36. Alatrash G, Hutson TE, Molto L, et al. Clinical and immunologic effects of subcutaneously administered interleukin-12 and inter-feron alfa-2b: phase I trial of patients with metastatic renal cell carcinoma or malignant melanoma. J Clin Oncol 2004;22(14): 2891–2900.
37. Kwon ED, Foster BA, Hurwitz AA, et al. Elimination of residual metastatic prostate cancer after surgery and adjunctive cytotoxic T lymphocyte-associated antigen 4 (CTLA-4) blockade immunother-apy. Proc Natl Acad Sci USA 1999;96(26):15074–15079.
38. Leach DR, Krummel MF, Allison JP. Enhancement of antitumor immunity by CTLA-4 blockade. Science 1996;271(5256):1734–1736.
39. Hodi FS, Mihm MC, Soiffer RJ, et al. Biologic activity of cytotoxic T lymphocyte-associated antigen 4 antibody blockade in previously vaccinated metastatic melanoma and ovarian carcinoma patients. Proc Natl Acad Sci USA 2003;100(8):4712–4717.
40. Escudier B, Lassau N, Couanet D, et al. Phase II trial of thalidomide in renal-cell carcinoma. Ann Oncol 2002;13(7):1029–1035.
41. Motzer RJ, Berg W, Ginsberg M, et al. Phase II trial of thalidomide for patients with advanced renal cell carcinoma. J Clin Oncol 2002;20(1):302–306.
42. Stebbing J, Benson C, Eisen T, et al. The treatment of advanced renal cell cancer with high-dose oral thalidomide. Br J Cancer 2001;85(7): 953–958.
43. Eisen T, Boshoff C, Mak I, et al. Continuous low dose thalidomide: a phase II study in advanced melanoma, renal cell, ovarian and breast cancer. Br J Cancer 2000;82(4):812–817.
44. Daliani DD, Papandreou CN, Thall PF, et al. A pilot study of thalido-mide in patients with progressive metastatic renal cell carcinoma. Cancer 2002;95(4):758–765.
45. Amato R, Breheny S, Tracy E. Phase I/II study of thalidomide + inter-leukin II (IL-2) for patients with metastatic renal cell carcinoma. Proc Am Soc Clin Oncol 2002;(abstr 759).
46. Rawat A, Amato RJ. Phase II Study of thalidomide, interleukin-2 (IL-2), and granulocyte macrophage-colony stimulating factor (GM-CSF) in patients with metastatic renal cell carcinoma (RCC). Proc Am Soc Clin Oncol 2004;(abstr 431).
47. Olencki T, Dreicer R, Elson P, Wood L, Bukowski R. Phase I trial of thalidomide and interleukin-2 (IL-2) in patients (pts) with metasta-tic renal cell carcinoma (RCC). Proc Am Soc Clin Oncol 2002;(abstr 2430).
48. Chapa P, Rawat A, Amato RJ. Phase II study of CC-5013 in patients (pts) with renal cell cancer (RCC). Proc Am Soc Clin Oncol 2004; (abstr 4761).

49. Gordon MS, Manola J, Fairclough D, et al. Low dose interferon-α2b (IFN) + thalidomide (T) in patients (pts) with previously untreated renal cell cancer (RCC). Improvement in progression-free survival (PFS) but not quality of life (QoL) or overall survival (OS). A phase III study of the Eastern Cooperative Oncology Group (E2898). Proc Am Soc Clin Oncol 2004;(abstr 4516).

50. Prescribing information, Pegasys package insert.

51. Prescribing information, Pegintron package insert.

52. Motzer RJ, Rakhit A, Thompson J, et al. II trial of branched peginterferon-alpha 2a (40 kDa) for patients with advanced renal cell carcinoma. Ann Oncol 2002;13(11):1799–1805.

53. Motzer RJ, Rakhit A, Ginsberg M, et al. Phase I trial of 40–kd branched pegylated interferon alfa-2a for patients with advanced renal cell carcinoma. J Clin Oncol 2001;19(5):1312–1319.

54. Bukowski R, Ernstoff MS, Gore ME, et al. Pegylated interferon alfa-2b treatment for patients with solid tumors: a phase I/II study. J Clin Oncol 2002;20(18):3841–3849.

55. Rosenberg SA, Lotze MT, Yang JC, et al. Prospective randomized trial of high-dose interleukin-2 alone or in conjunction with lymphokine-activated killer cells for the treatment of patients with advanced cancer. J Natl Cancer Inst 1993;85(8):622–632.

56. Law TM, Motzer RJ, Mazumdar M, et al. Phase III randomized trial of interleukin-2 with or without lymphokine-activated killer cells in the treatment of patients with advanced renal cell carcinoma. Cancer 1995;76(5):824–832.

57. Figlin RA, Thompson JA, Bukowski RM, et al. Multicenter, randomized, phase III trial of CD8(+) tumor-infiltrating lymphocytes in combination with recombinant interleukin-2 in metastatic renal cell carcinoma. J Clin Oncol 1999;17(8):2521–2529.

58. http://www.nci.nih.gov/search/clinical_trials/ (Search kidney cancer: STLMC-BRM-9401, NCI-V94–0514; John Hanson, P.I.).

59. Su Z, Dannull J, Heiser A, et al. Immunological and clinical responses in metastatic renal cancer patients vaccinated with tumor RNA-transfected dendritic cells. Cancer Res 2003;63(9):2127–2133.

60. Hirschowitz EA, Foody T, Kryscio R, Dickson L, Sturgill J, Yannelli J. Autologous dendritic cell vaccines for non-small-cell lung cancer. J Clin Oncol 2004;22(14):2808–2815.

61. Avigan D, Vasir B, Gong J, et al. Fusion cell vaccination of patients with metastatic breast and renal cancer induces immunological and clinical responses. Clin Cancer Res 2004;10(14):4699–4708.

62. Childs R, Chernoff A, Contentin N, et al. Regression of metastatic renal-cell carcinoma after nonmyeloablative allogeneic peripheral-blood stem-cell transplantation. N Engl J Med 2000;343(11):750–758.

63. Ueno NT, Cheng YC, Rondon G, et al. Rapid induction of complete donor chimerism by the use of a reduced-intensity conditioning regimen composed of fludarabine and melphalan in allogeneic stem

cell transplantation for metastatic solid tumors. Blood 2003;102(10): 3829–3836.

64. Blaise D, Bay JO, Faucher C, et al. Reduced-intensity preparative regimen and allogeneic stem cell transplantation for advanced solid tumors. Blood 2004;103(2):435–441.

65. Rini BI, Zimmerman TM, Gajewski TF, Stadler WM, Vogelzang NJ. Allogeneic peripheral blood stem cell transplantation for metastatic renal cell carcinoma. J Urol 2001;165(4):1208–1209.

66. Dai J, Liu B, Caudill MM, et al. Cell surface expression of heat shock protein gp96 enhances cross-presentation of cellular antigens and the generation of tumor-specific T cell memory. Cancer Immunol 2003;3:1.

67. Graner MW, Zeng Y, Feng H, Katsanis E. Tumor-derived chaperone-rich cell lysates are effective therapeutic vaccines against a variety of cancers. Cancer Immunol Immunother 2003;52(4):226–234.

68. Mazzaferro V, Coppa J, Carrabba MG, et al. Vaccination with autologous tumor-derived heat-shock protein gp96 after liver resection for metastatic colorectal cancer. Clin Cancer Res 2003;9(9):3235–3245.

69. http://www.antigenics.com/products/cancer/oncophage/ and http://www.antigenics.com/.

70. Antonia SJ, Seigne J, Diaz J, et al. Phase I trial of a B7-1 (CD80) gene modified autologous tumor cell vaccine in combination with systemic interleukin-2 in patients with metastatic renal cell carcinoma. J Urol 2002;167(5):1995–2000.

71. Borrello I, Sotomayor EM, Cooke S, Levitsky HI. A universal granulocyte-macrophage colony-stimulating factor-producing bystander cell line for use in the formulation of autologous tumor cell-based vaccines. Hum Gene Ther 1999;10(12):1983–1991.

72. http://www.gvax.com/home.shtml.

73. Jocham D, Richter A, Hoffmann L, et al. Adjuvant autologous renal tumour cell vaccine and risk of tumour progression in patients with renal-cell carcinoma after radical nephrectomy: phase III, randomised controlled trial. Lancet 2004;363(9409):594–599.

74. Fishman M, Antonia S. Specific antitumour vaccine for renal cancer. Lancet 2004;363(9409):583–584.

75. Folkman J, Kalluri R. Cancer without disease. Nature 2004;427(6977): 787.

76. Folkman J. Angiogenesis inhibitors: a new class of drugs. Cancer Biol Ther 2003;2(4 suppl 1):S127–133.

77. Nakamura M, Abe Y, Tokunaga T. Pathological significance of vascular endothelial growth factor A isoform expression in human cancer. Pathol Int 2002;52(5–6):331–339.

78. Clauss M. Molecular biology of the VEGF and the VEGF receptor family. Semin Thromb Hemost 2000;26(5):561–569.

79. Hurwitz H, Fehrenbacher L, Novotny W, et al. Bevacizumab plus irinotecan, fluorouracil, and leucovorin for metastatic colorectal cancer. N Engl J Med 2004;350(23):2335–2342.

80. Holash J, Davis S, Papadopoulos N, et al. VEGF-Trap: a VEGF blocker with potent antitumor effects. Proc Natl Acad Sci USA 2002; 99(17):11393–11398.

81. Yang JC, Haworth L, Sherry RM, et al. A randomized trial of bevacizumab, an anti-vascular endothelial growth factor antibody, for metastatic renal cancer. N Engl J Med 2003;349(5):427–434.

82. Rini BI, Halabi S, Taylor J, Small EJ, Schilsky RL. Cancer and Leukemia Group B 90206: a randomized phase III trial of interferon-alpha or interferon-alpha plus anti-vascular endothelial growth factor antibody (bevacizumab) in metastatic renal cell carcinoma. Clin Cancer Res 2004;10(8):2584–2586.

83. www.oxigene.com.

84. Stevenson JP, Rosen M, Sun W, et al. Phase I trial of the antivascular agent combretastatin A4 phosphate on a 5–day schedule to patients with cancer: magnetic resonance imaging evidence for altered tumor blood flow. J Clin Oncol 2003;21(23):4428–4438.

85. Thorpe PE. Vascular targeting agents as cancer therapeutics. Clin Cancer Res 2004;10(2):415–427.

86. Gingras D, Renaud A, Mousseau N, Beaulieu E, Kachra Z, Beliveau R. Matrix proteinase inhibition by AE-941, a multifunctional antiangiogenic compound. Anticancer Res 2001;21(1A):145–155.

87. Beliveau R, Gingras D, Kruger EA, et al. The antiangiogenic agent neovastat (AE-941) inhibits vascular endothelial growth factor-mediated biological effects. Clin Cancer Res 2002;8(4):1242–1250.

9

Chemotherapy for Testicular Cancer

Thomas R. Geldart and Graham M. Mead

Key Points

1. BEP is the standard treatment for metastatic disease.
2. Adjuvant treatment with carboplatin is a significant option for patients with seminoma.
3. Cure rates approach 98% for good prognosis teratoma and seminoma.

Introduction

The last 30 years have seen extraordinary advances in the management of metastatic germ cell cancer of the testis. Prior to the advent of cisplatin-containing chemotherapy in the mid-1970s, chemotherapy was highly toxic, and gave poor results, with cure unusual in those with advanced disease. Following the introduction of cisplatin, and subsequently etoposide, progress has been rapid, not least in the development of ancillary drugs (e.g., 5-hydroxytryptamine [5-HT$_3$] antagonists and growth factors). Modern therapy is now usually curative, tolerable, and has few long-term side effects. Indeed, the current dearth of randomized trials for most subgroups of these patients is largely a testimony to the advances taking place during this period.

This chapter describes the evolution of this therapy to the present, virtually worldwide consensus, emphasizing data derived from randomized trials. It is assumed throughout that patients with nonseminomatous germ cell cancer and residual masses postchemotherapy will, wherever possible, have these resected surgically. The emphasis is on failure-free survival and survival, the preferred trial end points in these diseases.

Prognostic Factors

Since the publication of the International Germ Cell Consensus Classification (IGCCC) data in 1997 [1], there has been virtually complete acceptance that patient management and clinical trials should be derived from the three prognostic groups of good, intermediate, and poor that were described in this study. Prior to this period, a wide variety of often conflicting parameters were used to allocate patients to two or three prognostic groups. It is beyond the scope of this text to describe each of these classifications in detail, and readers are referred to the original publications in each of the references for further detail.

In most modern studies, patients with seminoma requiring chemotherapy (a minority group) are combined with those with nonseminoma. Patients with seminoma are a median of 10 years older than patients with nonseminoma, which may have important implications for therapy. Those few studies specifically design for seminoma are considered separately.

Bleomycin, Etoposide, and Cisplatin (BEP): The Evolution of a Standard Therapy

The first effective steps in the development of effective chemotherapy for metastatic testicular cancer were the combination of vinblastine with infusional bleomycin and then incorporation of cisplatin to form the PVB regimen [2]. The Royal Marsden Hospital substituted etoposide (at a dose of $360\,mg/m^2$ given over 3 days per course) for vinblastine, resulting in the "European BEP" or BEP[360] regimen given for four courses at 3 weekly intervals, resulting in a highly effective regimen that became widely adopted in the United Kingdom [3]. International acceptance of BEP was to come when the Indiana Group, in a seminal study across all prognostic groups, compared four cycles of PVB and BEP^{500} (etoposide and cisplatin given over 5 days with etoposide at a total dose of 500 mg/m^2) [4]. A total of 244 evaluable patients were randomized, and BEP^{500} was found to improve survival in the poor prognostic group and to be associated with much improved tolerance. Bleomycin, given to a total dose of 360,000 IU in both arms resulted in five toxic deaths from bleomycin lung, and six patients died of infectious complications. Since this study was published, BEP, in many guises, has dominated the international therapy of metastatic germ cell cancer. Multiple attempts have been made to reduce its toxicity in patients with a good prognosis, and many studies have used BEP as a comparison against more intensive regimens in patients with a poor prognosis. These studies will now be described.

Treatment of Metastatic Disease

Good Prognosis Disease

Substitution of Carboplatin for Cisplatin

Platinum analogues have been one of the key elements in the successful evolution of germ cell cancer chemotherapy. Cisplatin is highly effective in combination, but universally associated with emesis, neurotoxicity, auditory toxicity, and renal toxicity. Carboplatin, although more myelotoxic, is associated with none of these problems and can be delivered easily on an outpatient basis. Initial studies suggested a high efficacy for this drug, particularly in seminoma (where it was widely adopted in Europe as a single agent for metastatic disease [5,6], but also in combination in nonseminoma [7], where comparative studies were designed to evaluate its role.

Seminoma

Two series from the Royal Marsden Hospital [5] and Germany [6] evaluated single-agent carboplatin in metastatic seminoma, both using a dose calculated from body surface area, rather than the more widely accepted area under the curve (AUC) dosing, giving 400 mg/m^2 of this drug every 3 to 4 weeks. The results from these two studies were remarkably similar, with failure-free survival rates of 71% and 77% and survival rates of 91% and 93%, respectively.

These two studies prompted two randomized trials (Table 9.1). The Medical Research Council (MRC) randomized 130 patients with metastatic seminoma between intravenous carboplatin and cisplatin/etoposide [8]. The trial was closed prematurely as recruitment had slowed following a negative assessment of carboplatin in metastatic nonseminoma in another trial. Carboplatin was associated with a 10% inferior progression-free survival (71% vs. 81%) with a nonsignificant survival difference favoring the cisplatin combination (84% vs. 89%). This study, however, was not adequately statistically powered.

A similar German study compared single-agent carboplatin against cisplatin, etoposide, and ifosfamide [9]. Published only in abstract form, the results were remarkably comparable (Table 9.1). A total of 280 patients were randomised, with 251 eligible for the study. Relapse-free survival favored the cisplatin-based combination (95% vs. 74%), although overall survival was not significantly different. It was recommended, as a result of this study, that carboplatin should not be used as a single agent in this setting. A subsequent meta-analysis evaluated data from the U.K., France, and Germany, and compared carboplatin- with cisplatin-containing drug combinations [10]. Data from 566 patients with seminoma was available. Once again progression-free survival for carboplatin was inferior (73% vs. 88% at 5 years) with no difference in survival (86% vs. 88%).

The authors of these studies felt unable to recommend single-agent carboplatin for general use in patients with metastatic seminoma. However, there can be no doubt that this treatment is occasionally useful in patients with seminoma unsuited to a more intensive cisplatin based schedule.

Nonseminoma/Mixed Populations (Table 9.2)

Two large studies have been reported comparing cisplatin against carboplatin combinations in this setting.

In a multiinstitutional study Bajorin et al. [11] compared cisplatin and etoposide given every 3 weeks against carboplatin (initially 350 mg/m^2 and then 500 mg/m^2) and etoposide given every

Table 9.1. Randomized trials in seminoma comparing carboplatin against cisplatin combinations

Author	Number	Median follow-up (months)	FFS (%)			Survival (%)			Comment
			Carbo	PEI	EP	Carbo	PEI	EP	
Horwich et al. (8)	130	54	71	—	81	84	—	89	Trial closed prematurely; NS differences; EC recommended
Clemm et al. (9)	280	52	74	95	—	87	95	—	Significant FFS benefit ($p = .01$); NS overall survival difference

FFS, failure-free survival; NS, nonsignificant; Carbo, carboplatin; PEI, cisplatin, etoposide, and ifosfamide; EC, etoposide and cisplatin.

Table 9.2. Randomized trials comparing cisplatin against carboplatin drug combinations in nonseminoma/mixed population

Author	Regimen	Number	FFS (%)	Survival (%)	Comment
Bajorin et al. (11)	EC	131	76	NS	EC inferior; comparable CR rate but more relapses
	EP	134	87	NS	
Horwich et al. (12)	CEB	260	77	90	Bleomycin given every 3 weeks; CEB significantly inferior
	BEP	268	91	97	

FFS, failure-free survival; NS, nonsignificant; EC, etoposide and carboplatin; EP, etoposide and cisplatin; CEB, carboplatin, etoposide and bleomycin; BEP, bleomycin, etoposide, and cisplatin.

4 weeks in a mixed seminoma/nonseminoma group with metastatic disease (Table 9.2). Twenty-two percent of randomised patients had seminoma. The study showed equivalent response rates and survival but inferior event-free survival for the carboplatin group, and it was concluded that carboplatin should be excluded from routine clinical use.

The MRC/European Organization for the Research and the Treatment of Cancer (EORTC) conducted a much larger, although comparable, study comparing European BEP[360] with BEC, substituting carboplatin at a dose of AUC 5 for cisplatin [12]. All patients in both arms received three weekly doses of bleomycin to a total dose of 120,000 IU intravenously. Failure-free survival and survival were inferior in the carboplatin arm (Table 9.2). However, it should be noted that the European BEP[360] arm delivered a creditable 97% 3-year survival.

There can be little doubt that carboplatin doses were less than ideal in the studies described above. In addition bleomycin was either omitted [11] or given at lower doses [12] than is conventional today. However, outside high-dose chemotherapy regimens and exceptional clinical circumstances, carboplatin is no longer used in the treatment of metastatic germ cell cancer.

Bleomycin: What Dose If Any? (Table 9.3)

Bleomycin is clearly a highly active drug in germ cell cancer. However, a 2% mortality rate and approximately 4% incidence of long-term dyspnea were repeatedly described in early studies. The Memorial Sloan-Kettering Cancer Center group has for many years omitted bleomycin from its treatment schedules for good prognosis testis cancer, preferring to rely on four cycles of EP (etoposide and cisplatin) [13], rather than three cycles of BEP, as has been widely adopted elsewhere. In a retrospective overview of its data in 195 patients, the group reported a compete response (CR) rate of 91% and a long-term survival rate of 86%, with even better results when a retrospectively derived IGCCC good prognosis group alone was evaluated [13].

Two randomised trials have directly evaluated the role of bleomycin in BEP (Table 9.3). De Wit and colleagues [14] from the EORTC randomised 419 good prognosis nonseminoma patients (using EORTC criteria) to European BEP[360] given with or without bleomycin (bleomycin total dose 360,000 IU). BEP was clearly more toxic, resulting in two deaths from bleomycin lung,

Table 9.3. BEP vs. EP in good prognosis seminoma

Author	Regimen	Number	FFS (%)	Survival (%)	Comment
De Wit et al. (14)	EP × 4	195	90	94	NS difference; 2 bleomycin related deaths in BEP arm; 4 vs. 8 cancer deaths BEP vs EP
	BEP × 4	200	93	97	
Loehrer et al. (15)	EP × 3	85	69	86	Significantly inferior FFS/survival in EP arm; study discontinued prematurely
	BEP × 3	86	86	95	

FFS, failure-free survival; NS, nonsignificant; EP, etoposide and cisplatin; BEP, bleomycin, etoposide, and Platinol (cisplatin).

a higher incidence of dyspnea, impaired pulmonary function, and all the cases of Raynaud's phenomenon. No significant differences were found in mortality (which was low), although there were more cancer-related deaths in the EP arm. They concluded that BEP was the treatment of choice, resulting in 10-year survival of 97%.

In a particularly fascinating study the Eastern Cooperative Oncology Group [15] randomized 178 patients with minimal or moderate metastatic disease (Indiana criteria) to three cycles of American BEP^{500} (bleomycin 270,000 IU), by then the standard treatment for this patient group (vide infra), versus three cycles of EP. The failure-free survival rates (86% vs. 69%) favored BEP and resulted from both a worse complete remission rate and a much higher relapse rate. Overall survival was less dramatically affected (91% vs. 86%) and not significantly different. Significant bleomycin toxicity was not seen in the BEP group. This study clearly indicated the threshold beneath which chemotherapy reduction can potentially cause loss of life. Further studies reducing therapy below three cycles of American BEP^{500} have not been initiated since this study report.

Number of Cycles of Treatment (Table 9.4)

From the early days in the development of platinum containing chemotherapy for germ cell cancer, four courses of chemotherapy (initially with PVB, later with BEP) were recommended. Following the development of effective prognostic factor classifications, new studies have attempted to reduce the number of chemotherapy courses in patients with a good prognosis, with the aim of reducing early and late treatment-related toxicity.

The first study in this group was published in 1989 from the South East Cancer Study Group (SECSG) [16]; subsequently cases entered from Indiana were updated in a separate publication in 1998 [17]. Patients with minimal or moderate extent (Indiana criteria) metastatic germ cell cancer were randomized to either three or four courses of American BEP^{500}. A total of 184 patients were randomised, and 92% in both arms remained failure free. This study was powered to show a 10% or greater reduction in response rates, and concerns were expressed about the potential size of an undetectable difference in efficacy.

In view of these concerns, a much larger EORTC-MRC trial was designed and implemented [18,19]. This used the then recently

Table 9.4. Comparison of number of BEP cycles in patients with good prognosis non-seminoma

Author	Regimen	Number	FFS (%)	Survival (%)	Comment
SECSG (16,17)	BEP × 3	88	92	91	NS difference; initial results updated at 10 years; 98% survival when HCG < 1000
	BEP × 4	96	92	93	
MRC/EORTC (18,19)	BEP × 3	406	90.4	97	Bleomycin total dose 270,000 IU all patients; NS difference between trial arms
	BEP × 3 EP × 1	406	89.4	97.1	
	BEP 3 day	339	88.8	96.4	
	BEP 5 day	342	89.7	97.5	

FFS, failure-free survival; NS, nonsignificant; EP, etoposide and cisplatin; BEP, bleomycin, etoposide, and cisplatin; HCG, human chorionic gonadotropin.

published IGCCC criteria for prognosis, incorporating the good prognosis group only. The study was designed as a 2×2 study comparing three against four cycles of BEP and also the administration of chemotherapy over either 3 or 5 days. A total of 812 patients were entered into the first randomisation and 681 into the second. The bleomycin dose was limited to 270,000 IU for all patients. The study showed no difference in progression-free survival between any of the four arms. A quality of life study published separately demonstrated increased gastrointestinal toxicity and tinnitus in patients receiving four cycles of chemotherapy over 3 rather than 5 days [19]. Otherwise no significant treatment differences were found.

Comparative BEP Regimen Studies (Table 9.5)

Two studies fit best into this group. The first compared four cycles of European BEP[360] with three weekly bleomycin doses, as described above [12], with three cycles of American BEP[500]. The study took place in Australasia, where both regimens were in widespread use at this time [20]. A comparative study was thereby deemed of interest.

A total of 166 patients of a planned 260 were randomized. The study used a modified Memorial Hospital New York, NY definition of good prognosis. Subsequent reanalyses using IGCCC criteria found 17% of patients had an intermediate or poor prognosis with an imbalanced excess randomisation to European BEP[360]. Recruitment was suspended after an interim analysis suggested superior survival for three cycles of American BEP[500]. Overall, significantly improved survival was apparent in this group with a total of one versus nine cancer-related deaths.

The second study in this group has this far been published only in abstract form [21]. This French study defined good prognosis using a mathematical model from the Institut Gustav Roussy and randomized 270 patients between three cycles of American BEP[500] and four cycles of the same regimen without bleomycin (EP). Adverse events (toxic death, relapse from favourable response, incomplete response, and surgical CR) occurred more commonly in the four-EP group such that 4-year event-free survival, (EFS), was 89% in the 3-BEP arm and 84% in the 4-EP arm ($p = .09$). Overall survival was not significantly different. The authors concluded that three cycles of BEP should be standard therapy.

Table 9.5. Comparative studies of BEP regimens

Author	Regimen	Number	FFS (%)	Survival (%)	Comment
Toner et al. (20)	BEP^{360} × 4 BEP^{500} × 3	83 83	77 81	84 96	Study discontinued prematurely; American BEP^{500} significantly better survival ($p = .008$)
Culine et al. (21)	BEP^{500} × 3 EP × 4	131 127	89 84	96 92	Significant failure-free survival advantage for American BEP^{500} ($p = .037$); no overall survival difference; American BEP^{500} better tolerated

FFS, failure-free survival; NS, nonsignificant; EP, etoposide and cisplatin; BEP^{360}, bleomycin, etoposide (360 mg/m^2 per cycle), and cisplatin; BEP^{500}, bleomycin, etoposide (500 mg/m^2 per cycle), and cisplatin.

Which BEP for Good Prognosis Disease?: Conclusions

The remarkable series of trials described above have effectively examined BEP in all its guises. The excellent outlook of patients with good prognosis disease in modern oncology practice (anticipated failure-free survival [FFS] 90% and overall survival 95% to 98%) make it almost impossible to construct a reasonable-sized trial to confirm the equivalence of any two regimens. A number of these trials have thereby reported number of "adverse events," that is, failure of therapy, resection of cancer postchemotherapy, or toxic death rather than overall difference in FFS. Although not entirely satisfactory, these analyses all point to three cycles of American BEP^{500} as the preferred standard therapy. This treatment should be easily delivered to a substantial proportion of patients, with alternatives (particularly EP × 4) reserved for those at increased risk of bleomycin lung toxicity by virtue of age or preceding lung or renal dysfunction. Carboplatin should rarely be used either as a single agent (seminoma) or in combination. However, despite inferior progression-free survival in seminoma and (probably) overall survival in nonseminoma, regimens containing this drug can still cure a majority of patients.

Intermediate Prognosis Disease

Only a single study has been designed for this IGCCC group. The EORTC/MRC have an ongoing study comparing standard American BEP^{500} (four cycles) with T-BEP (BEP^{500} given together with paclitaxel at a dose of 175 mg/m^2 per course) supported by filgrastim. This study has completed an initial phase II evaluation, and subject to the results has now proceeded to a phase III trial.

Poor Prognosis Disease (Table 9.6)

This is a comparatively uncommon group, and trial accrual has historically been slow. In general, studies in this group have used four cycles of American BEP^{500} as a control, comparing this with a more intensive treatment in the remaining arm of the study.

In an early intergroup study from Indiana University, 159 patients with advanced metastatic disease by Indiana criteria were randomised to receive four cycles of American BEP^{500} or the same regimen with double-dose cisplatin (40 mg/m^2 IV daily for

Table 9.6. Randomized studies in poor prognosis disease

Group	Regimen	Number	FFS (%)	Survival (%)	Comment
SWOG (22)	BEP[20]	78	61	74	NS difference; markedly increased toxicity with high-dose cisplatin arm
	BEP[40]	76	63	74	
Intergroup (23,24)	BEP[500] × 4	139	58	67	Updated results ≥7 year follow-up; NS difference; BEP arm less toxic and recommended
	VIP × 4	142	64	69	
MRC/EORTC (25)	BEP[500]/EP × 6	190	60	76	NS difference; BEP/EP less toxic and recommended
	BOP/VIP-B	190	53	71	

FFS, failure-free survival; NS, nonsignificant; EP, etoposide and cisplatin; BEP[500], bleomycin, etoposide (500 mg/m^2 per cycle), and cisplatin; VIP, etoposide, ifosfamide, and cisplatin; BOP/VIP-B, bleomycin, vincristine, cisplatin, etopside, ifosfamide.

5 days) [22]. This modest-sized trial was designed to detect a 20% improvement in outcome but failed to do so. At the time of analysis the results from the two arms were essentially identical (Table 9.6). Cisplatin dose escalation resulted in unacceptable neurotoxicity and has not been used since this study.

In a second and larger intergroup trial of 304 patients with advanced stage GCT (Indiana criteria), four cycles of BEP[500] were compared with four cycles of VIP (etoposide, ifosfamide, and cisplatin) [23]. This study was initially published in 1998 and subsequently updated in 2003 [24]. Remarkably at the time of the update and after reclassification of prognostic factors, 36% of the patients were found to have an IGCCC good or intermediate prognosis rather than a poor prognosis. This study showed no significant benefit from the use of the more myelotoxic VIP regimen in any patient group but did demonstrate that this regimen was an effective alternative when doubts about bleomycin pulmonary toxicity existed.

The MRC and EORTC have also conducted a trial in patients with poor prognosis disease incorporating 380 patients and using MRC/EORTC prognostic factor data [25] (Table 9.6). The trial randomised patients to receive six cycles of American BEP[500]/EP[500] or six cycles of BOP/VIP-B, comprising an initial dose-intense induction with bleomycin, vincristine, and cisplatin given every 10 days, followed by three cycles of VIP with bleomycin. As in the American VIP study, when patients were reclassified by IGCCC criteria 39% fell into the good/intermediate prognosis group. No significant difference was detected between BEP[500] and BOP/VIP-B, with 1-year FFS rates in the two original groups of 60% (BEP/EP) and 53% BOP/VIP-B. A subset of patients in this trial were also randomised to filgrastim or no growth factor support [26]. This study showed that filgrastim increased the ability to deliver full-dose chemotherapy and also reduced treatment-related mortality in the BOP/VIP-B arm. However, no benefit was seen in the patients receiving BEP[500]/EP[500], and filgrastim support was not recommended for patients receiving BEP in the future.

In an additional analysis, the EORTC evaluated the impact on survival of patients in the study by treating institution [27]. Patients entered into the study from centers accruing fewer than five patients had worse survival than did patients from those centers entering more patients ($p = .01$, hazard ratio 1.85). The data suggested that the underlying reasons were the less intensive treatment delivery and less surgical intervention post-chemotherapy at the smaller treatment centers.

Nonrandomized Trials and Ongoing Phase III Trials

There are currently no large randomized trials in progress in patients with good prognosis metastatic germ cell cancer. For patients with intermediate prognosis disease, the EORTC is currently comparing BEP with T-BEP (see above).

In patients with poor prognosis disease, two main approaches have been tested in phase II trials and are currently undergoing phase III evaluation. High-dose therapy with autologous bone marrow support is one such approach that was initially introduced as a salvage therapy. The achievement of cure in some heavily pretreated patients (in conjunction with the advent of peripheral stem cell harvest and the development of growth factors) has led to the application of this approach in poor prognostic group patients early in their disease course [28]. In a our U.S. intergroup study, patients with poor prognosis teratoma were randomized between four cycles of American BEP^{500} versus two cycles of BEP^{500} and two cycles of high-dose chemotherapy with peripheral stem cell support. Trial analysis is awaited.

In Europe, a slightly different approach has been developed, initially in Germany [29,30]. Following an initial cycle of VIP and stem cell harvest, three further cycles of this chemotherapy are given at high dose (etoposide 1.5 g/m^2, ifosfamide 10 g/m^2, and cisplatin 100 mg/m^2) over 5 days at three weekly intervals with growth factor and stem cell support. This regimen is currently being randomised against four cycles of American BEP^{500} in an EORTC study.

Two further treatment regimens warrant mention: POMB ACE [31] and C-BOP BEP [32] are intensive cycling regimens devised in the U.K. and predominantly evaluated in intermediate/poor prognosis patients. Both have produced impressive results in a single institution setting, but to date neither has been evaluated in randomized trials.

Which BEP for Intermediate/Poor Prognosis Disease?

Patients with intermediate or poor prognosis disease should always be classified using IGCCC criteria. No comparative evaluation of BEP regimens or numbers of treatment courses have been carried out in this group. Wherever possible patients should be treated in large treatment centers with a specialist interested in germ cell cancers, and should be entered into randomized trials where these are available. World standard therapy for this group still remains four cycles of American BEP[500]. Many clinicians prefer to restrict the total bleomycin dose to 270,000 IU in this subgroup as well as in patients with a good prognosis, particularly if patients are to go on to receive abdominal or thoracic surgery after induction chemotherapy. The results of the EORTC and American randomized trials described above are awaited with interest.

Adjuvant Chemotherapy

Following the development of effective chemotherapy regimens for the treatment of metastatic germ cell cancer, a number of studies have gone on to evaluate the role of chemotherapy in the adjuvant setting following surgery for stage I disease.

Nonseminomatous Germ Cell Cancer

Approximately 40% of men presenting with testicular nonseminomatous germ cell cancer have stage I disease (normal staging on a computed tomography [CT] scan, normal tumor markers, or markers that normalize following orchidectomy) with an anticipated risk of systemic relapse of 25% for patients followed by surveillance. Histopathological examination of the resected testis enables stratification of patients with stage I disease into two groups at low or at high risk of relapse. Combined data from MRC surveillance studies have shown that lymphovascular invasion by tumor is the major risk factor for relapse [33,34]. Its identification (in approximately 25% of orchidectomy specimens) predicts a increased risk of relapse in the order of 40%.

Risk adapted adjuvant treatment in patients with high-risk stage I nonseminomatous germ cell cancer has been evaluated in a number of small studies and one large prospective trial conducted by the MRC [35–40]. The MRC trial prospectively evaluated the efficacy and long-term toxicity of two cycles of BEP[360] chemotherapy in 114 high-risk patients. After a median follow-up of 4 years, the relapse-free rate at 2 years was 98%, substantially less than the 40% to 50% relapse rate predicted by previous studies of surveillance [33,34]. Clinically significant long-term toxicity was not encountered in this study, although individuals will have been exposed to significant short-term side effects (e.g., myelosuppression, alopecia, nausea). It is noteworthy that although adjuvant BEP[360] chemotherapy may substantially reduce an individual's risk of relapse, 60% of high-risk patients are cured by surgery alone and therefore receive chemotherapy unnecessarily. Moreover, patients managed by surveillance who develop systemic disease almost invariably relapse with good prognosis disease, and for such patients three cycles of BEP results in failure-free survival of at least 90% [1]. Therefore, the use of adjuvant chemotherapy in stage I nonseminomatous testicular cancer should remain a matter of choice for patients.

Testicular Seminoma

For men presenting with stage I testicular seminoma, surveillance studies demonstrate that approximately 15–20% of individuals relapse systemically following orchidectomy and go on to require radiotherapy or systemic chemotherapy treatment for metastatic disease [41]. Relapse may occur late and is less commonly associated with tumor marker elevation than nonseminomatous tumors. As such, surveillance relies heavily on prolonged radiological (CT) follow-up and is not commonly used.

Radiotherapy has been shown to decrease the risk of relapse and has remained standard adjuvant therapy for this group of patients for many years. A number of MRC randomized clinical trials have focused on decreasing both the extent (TE10) [42] and dose (TE18) [43] of radiotherapy. On the basis of these trials, the current practice is to treat patients with para-aortic nodal strip radiotherapy at a dose of 20 Gy in 10 fractions over 2 weeks, with an expected 3-year failure-free survival of 96%.

Although the use of radiotherapy is effective in reducing the risk of systemic relapse, treatment is associated with a small but definite increase in second malignancies [44,45]. Metastatic seminoma is an extremely chemosensitive disease, and with the aim of reducing treatment-related morbidity, a number of phase II trials have evaluated the use of single-agent carboplatin as an alternative approach to adjuvant therapy for this patient group [46–49]. These early trials suggested carboplatin to be a well-tolerated and effective adjuvant therapy, and as such, a confirmatory, prospective MRC phase III trial was set up to formally compare a single dose of carboplatin (AUC 7) against adjuvant para-aortic strip radiotherapy. A total of 1477 patients were recruited into this trial, which closed to recruitment in March 2001. A median follow-up of 3 years has now elapsed, and preliminary results were presented in abstract form at the American Society of Clinical Oncology (ASCO) 2004 meeting. This trial has shown that adjuvant radiotherapy and carboplatin are of equivalent efficacy. Carboplatin can thereby be regarded as an equivalent (and probably preferred) management approach.

Long-Term Toxicities of Chemotherapy for Germ Cell Cancers

The majority of patients with testicular germ cell cancer are cured by surgery alone or surgery in combination with cisplatin-based chemotherapy and/or radiotherapy. In general, patients cured of their disease have a long life expectancy, and therefore the potential long-term toxicities of treatment are of considerable importance. A number of studies have evaluated the long-term toxicities of platinum-based chemotherapy.

Fertility and Gonadal Function

Spermatogenesis is impaired in a substantial proportion of patients presenting with germ cell cancer. In normospermic men who undergo combination BEP chemotherapy, a reduction in fertility is apparent postchemotherapy, although for most individuals sperm counts will recover over a period of years [50]. Of note, a good prechemotherapy sperm count is associated with a increased likelihood of recovery of spermatogenesis. With regard to hormonal function, a comparison of patients treated with surgery alone or surgery plus chemotherapy suggests that standard-dose BEP chemotherapy does not seem to contribute additionally to a significant impairment in Leydig cell function [51]. In contrast, higher doses ($\geq$400 mg/m^2 cisplatin) may be associated with a significant and persistent impact in Leydig cell function with a consequent reduction in mean testosterone levels.

Pulmonary Function

As discussed earlier, the use of bleomycin has long been associated with pulmonary toxicity, with studies recording a 4% to 6% incidence of demonstrable lung toxicity with a 1% to 2%

mortality rate. Toxicity is predominantly fibrotic in nature. Standard lung function tests are generally unhelpful in predicting toxicity and treatments (such as steroids) for established toxicity of unproven benefit. A number of pretreatment parameters do predict for bleomycin-induced toxicity, and these include poor renal function, age greater than 40, cumulative bleomycin dose greater than 300,000 units, and stage IV disease [52]. Careful consideration of bleomycin dose and close monitoring of patients presenting with one or more of these risk factors is of considerable importance.

Cardiovascular Morbidity

A number of studies have suggested a higher than expected incidence of cardiovascular disease (CVD) in patients receiving chemotherapy for metastatic disease. The largest of these studies has suggested that after a median of 10 years' follow-up, there may be a twofold or greater risk of developing CVD in such patients when compared to (stage I) matched patients followed by surveillance alone; the absolute risk is 6.7%, and the age-adjusted relative risk is 2.59 (95% confidence interval [CI], 1.1 to 5.8) [53]. A variety of potential mechanisms could ac-count for an increased risk of CVD following chemotherapy, including vascular endothelial damage, renal impairment, hypertension, hyperlipidemia, and an increase in body mass index. Although no clear relationship was established for any of these risk factors in this study, other studies have demonstrated a relationship between chemotherapy and an increased incidence of classical CVD risk factors such as plasma lipid profiles and raised blood pressure [54].

Secondary Malignancies

Large population-based studies have suggested a small but significant increase in the subsequent risk of acute leukemia in patients who have received cisplatin/etoposide-based chemotherapy for metastatic testicular cancer. The risk appears to be dose related, but for conventional dose treatment (three to four cycles of BEP), the relative risk may be increased by approximately threefold or more [55]. However, it is noteworthy that in absolute values, this translates to an extremely small increase in incidence in the region of 1.6 per 1000 patients treated. Clearly, the huge survival advantage provided by chemotherapy far outweighs this small absolute risk of a secondary leukemia.

Neuropathy

Cisplatin-induced sensory neuropathy is commonly encountered following BEP chemotherapy. Approximately 15% to 20% of individuals experience persisting neuropathy following treatment, with prevalence, severity, and duration of neuropathy being related to increasing cisplatin dose [56]. Additionally, persistent symptomatic ototoxicity (manifested by high-tone hearing loss and tinnitus) may been seen in approximately 20% receiving standard-dose BEP chemotherapy with prevalence increasing to around 60% in those patients receiving higher (≥600 mg) cumulative doses of cisplatin [57]. Following completion of chemotherapy, cisplatin-induced neuropathy and ototoxicity generally improve over time and may resolve completely for a substantial number of individuals. However, severe neuropathy related to high cumulative doses of cisplatin may persist long term.

Conclusion

The last 30 years has seen a revolution in the chemotherapy treatment of germ cell cancer, and the vast majority of patients with metas-tatic disease can now expect to be cured. Worldwide, BEP remains the gold standard chemotherapy treatment for all groups of patients presenting with metastatic germ cell cancer. For patients presenting with good prognosis metastatic disease, cure rates now approach 98% and the research focus has switched from improving outcome to reducing treatment-related morbidity. For patients with intermediate and poor prognosis metastatic disease, further improvements in treatment outcomes remain a research priority through the use of novel agents or the safe delivery of dose-intensified treatments. In the adjuvant setting, short-course BEP has established itself as a treatment option for high-risk stage I nonseminoma; for seminoma, the use of single-agent carboplatin seems likely to replace para-aortic nodal strip radiotherapy as the standard adjuvant treatment for stage I disease. The long-term morbidities of BEP chemotherapy are now more clearly defined and allow for an informed discussion with patients about to embark on chemotherapy and appropriate surveillance of individuals thereafter. It would be optimistic to predict that the next 30 years will yield as many advances in the treatment of this disease as have been witnessed since the mid-1970s; however, with our ever-increasing understanding about the natural history and biology of this disease, we should remain determined in our efforts to maximize cure and minimize morbidity in all patients presenting with germ cell cancer.

Controversies and Outstanding Issues

1. Can we identify curative treatment for patients with recurrent or non responsive tumours?
2. Is research morally and ethically possible in a disease where cure rates are>95%?

References

1. International Germ Cell Cancer Collaborative Group. International Germ Cell Consensus Classification: a prognostic factor-based staging system for metastatic germ cell cancers. J Clin Oncol 1997; 15(2):594–603.
2. Einhorn LH, Donohue J. Cis-diamminedichloroplatinum, vinblastine, and bleomycin combination chemotherapy in disseminated testicular cancer. Ann Intern Med 1977;87(3):293–298.
3. Peckham MJ, Barrett A, Liew KH, et al. The treatment of metastatic germ-cell testicular tumours with bleomycin, etoposide and cisplatin (BEP). Br J Cancer 1983;47(5):613–619.
4. Williams SD, Birch R, Einhorn LH, Irwin L, Greco FA, Loehrer PJ. Treatment of disseminated germ-cell tumors with cisplatin, bleomycin, and either vinblastine or etoposide. N Engl J Med 1987;316(23):1435–1440.
5. Horwich A, Dearnaley DP, A'Hern R, et al. The activity of single-agent carboplatin in advanced seminoma. Eur J Cancer 1992;28A(8–9): 1307–1310.
6. Schmoll HJ, Harstrick A, Bokemeyer C, et al. Single-agent carboplatinum for advanced seminoma. A phase II study. Cancer 1993;72(1):237–243.
7. Childs WJ, Nicholls EJ, Horwich A. The optimisation of carboplatin dose in carboplatin, etoposide and bleomycin combination chemotherapy for good prognosis metastatic nonseminomatous germ cell tumours of the testis. Ann Oncol 1992;3(4):291–296.

8. Horwich A, Oliver RT, Wilkinson PM, et al. A medical research council randomized trial of single agent carboplatin versus etoposide and cisplatin for advanced metastatic seminoma. MRC Testicular Tumour Working Party. Br J Cancer 2000;83(12):1623–1629.

9. Clemm C, Bokemeyer C, Gerl A, et al. Randomized trial comparing cisplatin/etoposide/ifosfamide with carboplatin monotherapy in patients with advanced metastatic seminoma. Proc Am Soc Clin Oncol 2000:326a.

10. Bokemeyer C, Kollmannsberger C, Flechon A, et al. Prognostic factors in patients (pts) with advanced metastatic seminoma (SEM) treated with either single agent carboplatin (CP) or cisplatin based (DDP) combination chemotherapy (CTX): a meta-analysis of prospective European trials. Proc Am Soc Clin Oncol 2002;19: 186a.

11. Bajorin DF, Sarosdy MF, Pfister DG, et al. Randomized trial of etoposide and cisplatin versus etoposide and carboplatin in patients with good-risk germ cell tumors: a multiinstitutional study. J Clin Oncol 1993;11(4):598–606.

12. Horwich A, Sleijfer DT, Fossa SD, et al. Randomized trial of bleomycin, etoposide, and cisplatin compared with bleomycin, etoposide, and carboplatin in good-prognosis metastatic nonseminomatous germ cell cancer: a Multiinstitutional Medical Research Council/European Organization for Research and Treatment of Cancer Trial. J Clin Oncol 1997;15(5):1844–1852.

13. Xiao H, Mazumdar M, Bajorin DF, et al. Long-term follow-up of patients with good-risk germ cell tumors treated with etoposide and cisplatin. J Clin Oncol 1997;15(7):2553–2558.

14. de Wit R, Stoter G, Kaye SB, et al. Importance of bleomycin in combination chemotherapy for good-prognosis testicular nonseminoma: a randomized study of the European Organization for Research and Treatment of Cancer Genitourinary Tract Cancer Cooperative Group. J Clin Oncol 1997;15(5):1837–1843.

15. Loehrer PJ Sr, Johnson D, Elson P, Einhorn LH, Trump D. Importance of bleomycin in favorable-prognosis disseminated germ cell tumors: an Eastern Cooperative Oncology Group trial. J Clin Oncol 1995; 13(2):470–476.

16. Einhorn LH, Williams SD, Loehrer PJ, et al. Evaluation of optimal duration of chemotherapy in favorable-prognosis disseminated germ cell tumors: a Southeastern Cancer Study Group protocol. J Clin Oncol 1989;7(3):387–391.

17. Saxman SB, Finch D, Gonin R, Einhorn LH. Long-term follow-up of a phase III study of three versus four cycles of bleomycin, etoposide, and cisplatin in favorable-prognosis germ-cell tumors: the Indian University experience. J Clin Oncol 1998;16(2):702–706.

18. de Wit R, Roberts JT, Wilkinson PM, et al. Equivalence of three or four cycles of bleomycin, etoposide, and cisplatin chemotherapy and of a 3- or 5-day schedule in good-prognosis germ cell cancer: a randomized study of the European Organization for Research and Treatment of Cancer Genitourinary Tract Cancer Cooperative Group and the Medical Research Council. J Clin Oncol 2001;19(6):1629–1640.

19. Fossa SD, de Wit R, Roberts JT, et al. Quality of life in good prognosis patients with metastatic germ cell cancer: a prospective study of the European Organization for Research and Treatment of Cancer Genitourinary Group/Medical Research Council Testicular Cancer Study Group (30941/TE20). J Clin Oncol 2003;21(6):1107–1118.

20. Toner GC, Stockler MR, Boyer MJ, et al. Comparison of two standard chemotherapy regimens for good-prognosis germ-cell tumours: a randomised trial. Australian and New Zealand Germ Cell Trial Group. Lancet 2001;357(9258):739–745.

21. Culine S, Kerbrat P, Bouzy J, et al. The optimal chemotherapy regimen for good-risk metastatic non seminomatous germ cell tumours (MSNGCT) is 3 cycles of bleomycin, etoposide and cisplatin. Mature results of a randomized trial. Proc Am Soc Clin Oncol 2003;22:382.

22. Nichols CR, Williams SD, Loehrer PJ, et al. Randomized study of cisplatin dose intensity in poor-risk germ cell tumors: a Southeastern Cancer Study Group and Southwest Oncology Group protocol. J Clin Oncol 1991;9(7):1163–1172.

23. Nichols CR, Catalano PJ, Crawford ED, Vogelzang NJ, Einhorn LH, Loehrer PJ. Randomized comparison of cisplatin and etoposide and either bleomycin or ifosfamide in treatment of advanced disseminated germ cell tumors: an Eastern Cooperative Oncology Group, Southwest Oncology Group, and Cancer and Leukemia Group B Study. J Clin Oncol 1998;16(4):1287–1293.

24. Hinton S, Catalano PJ, Einhorn LH, et al. Cisplatin, etoposide and either bleomycin or ifosfamide in the treatment of disseminated germ cell tumors: final analysis of an intergroup trial. Cancer 2003;97(8):1869–1875.

25. Kaye SB, Mead GM, Fossa S, et al. Intensive induction-sequential chemotherapy with BOP/VIP-B compared with treatment with BEP/EP for poor-prognosis metastatic nonseminomatous germ cell tumor: a randomized Medical Research Council/European Organization for Research and Treatment of Cancer study. J Clin Oncol 1998;16(2):692–701.

26. Fossa SD, Kaye SB, Mead GM, et al. Filgrastim during combination chemotherapy of patients with poor-prognosis metastatic germ cell malignancy. European Organization for Research and Treatment of Cancer, Genito-Urinary Group, and the Medical Research Council Testicular Cancer Working Party, Cambridge, United Kingdom. J Clin Oncol 1998;16(2):716–724.

27. Collette L, Sylvester RJ, Stenning SP, et al. Impact of the treating institution on survival of patients with "poor-prognosis" metastatic non-seminoma. European Organization for Research and Treatment of Cancer Genito-Urinary Tract Cancer Collaborative Group and the Medical Research Council Testicular Cancer Working Party. J Natl Cancer Inst 1999;91(10):839–846.

28. Motzer RJ, Mazumdar M, Bajorin DF, Bosl GJ, Lyn P, Vlamis V. High-dose carboplatin, etoposide, and cyclophosphamide with autologous bone marrow transplantation in first-line therapy for patients with poor-risk germ cell tumors. J Clin Oncol 1997;15(7): 2546–2552.

29. Bokemeyer C, Schmoll HJ, Harstrick A, et al. A phase I/II study of a stepwise dose-escalated regimen of cisplatin, etoposide and ifosfamide plus granulocyte-macrophage colony-stimulating factor (GM-CSF) in patients with advanced germ cell tumours. Eur J Cancer 1993;29A(16):2225–2231.

30. Schmoll HJ, Kollmannsberger C, Metzner B, et al. Long-term results of first-line sequential high-dose etoposide, ifosfamide, and cisplatin chemotherapy plus autologous stem cell support for patients with advanced metastatic germ cell cancer: an extended phase I/II study of the German Testicular Cancer Study Group. J Clin Oncol 2003;21(22):4083–4091.

31. Bower M, Newlands ES, Holden L, Rustin GJ, Begent RH. Treatment of men with metastatic non-seminomatous germ cell tumours with cyclical POMB/ACE chemotherapy. Ann Oncol 1997;8(5):477–483.

32. Christian JA, Huddart RA, Norman A, et al. Intensive induction chemotherapy with CBOP/BEP in patients with poor prognosis germ cell tumors. J Clin Oncol 2003;21(5):871–877.

33. Freedman LS, Parkinson MC, Jones WG, et al. Histopathology in the prediction of relapse of patients with stage I testicular teratoma treated by orchidectomy alone. Lancet 1987;2(8554):294–298.

34. Read G, Stenning SP, Cullen MH, et al. Medical Research Council prospective study of surveillance for stage I testicular teratoma. Medical Research Council Testicular Tumors Working Party. J Clin Oncol 1992;10(11):1762–1768.

35. Bohlen D, Borner M, Sonntag RW, Fey MF, Studer UE. Long-term results following adjuvant chemotherapy in patients with clinical stage I testicular nonseminomatous malignant germ cell tumors with high risk factors. J Urol 1999;161(4):1148–1152.

36. Oliver RT, Raja MA, Ong J, Gallagher CJ. Pilot study to evaluate impact of a policy of adjuvant chemotherapy for high risk stage 1 malignant teratoma on overall relapse rate of stage 1 cancer patients. J Urol 1992;148(5):1453–1455; discussion 1455–1456.

37. Pont J, Albrecht W, Postner G, Sellner F, Angel K, Holtl W. Adjuvant chemotherapy for high-risk clinical stage I nonseminomatous

testicular germ cell cancer: long-term results of a prospective trial. J Clin Oncol 1996;14(2):441–448.

38. Cullen MH, Stenning SP, Parkinson MC, et al. Short-course adjuvant chemotherapy in high-risk stage I nonseminomatous germ cell tumors of the testis: a Medical Research Council report. J Clin Oncol 1996;14(4):1106–1113.

39. Abratt RP, Pontin AR, Barnes RD, Reddi BV. Adjuvant chemotherapy for stage I non-seminomatous testicular cancer. S Afr Med J 1994;84(9):605–607.

40. Studer UE, Burkhard FC, Sonntag RW. Risk adapted management with adjuvant chemotherapy in patients with high risk clinical stage I nonseminomatous germ cell tumor. J Urol 2000;163(6):1785–1787.

41. Warde P, Gospodarowicz MK, Banerjee D, et al. Prognostic factors for relapse in stage I testicular seminoma treated with surveillance. J Urol 1997;157(5):1705–1709; discussion 1709–1710.

42. Fossa SD, Horwich A, Russell JM, et al. Optimal planning target volume for stage I testicular seminoma: A Medical Research Council randomized trial. Medical Research Council Testicular Tumor Working Group. J Clin Oncol 1999;17(4):1146.

43. Jones WG, Fossa SD, Mead GM, et al. A randomised trial of two radio-therapy schedules in the adjuvant treatment of stage I seminoma (MRC TE18). Eur J Cancer 2001;37(suppl 6):S157.

44. van Leeuwen FE, Stiggelbout AM, van den Belt-Dusebout AW, et al. Second cancer risk follow-ing testicular cancer: a follow-up study of 1,909 patients. J Clin Oncol 1993;11(3):415–424.

45. Wanderas EH, Fossa SD, Tretli S. Risk of subsequent non-germ cell cancer after treatment of germ cell cancer in 2006 Norwegian male patients. Eur J Cancer 1997;33(2):253–262.

46. Dieckmann KP, Bruggeboes B, Pichlmeier U, Kuster J, Mullerleile U, Bartels H. Adjuvant treatment of clinical stage I seminoma: is a single course of carboplatin sufficient? Urology 2000;55(1):102–106.

47. Aparicio J, Garcia del Muro X, Maroto P, et al. Multicenter study eval-uating a dual policy of postorchiectomy surveillance and selective adjuvant single-agent carboplatin for patients with clinical stage I seminoma. Ann Oncol 2003;14(6):867–872.

48. Krege S, Kalund G, Otto T, Goepel M, Rubben H. Phase II study: adju-vant single-agent carboplatin therapy for clinical stage I seminoma. Eur Urol 1997;31(4):405–407.

49. Oliver RT, Edmonds PM, Ong JY, et al. Pilot studies of 2 and 1 course carboplatin as adjuvant for stage I seminoma: should it be tested in a randomized trial against radiotherapy? Int J Radiat Oncol Biol Phys 1994;29(1):3–8.

50. Lampe H, Horwich A, Norman A, Nicholls J, Dearnaley DP. Fertility after chemotherapy for testicular germ cell cancers. J Clin Oncol 1997;15(1):239–245.

51. Gerl A, Muhlbayer D, Hansmann G, Mraz W, Hiddemann W. The impact of chemotherapy on Leydig cell function in long term survivors of germ cell tumors. Cancer 2001;91(7):1297–1303.
52. O'Sullivan JM, Huddart RA, Norman AR, Nicholls J, Dearnaley DP, Horwich A. Predicting the risk of bleomycin lung toxicity in patients with germ-cell tumours. Ann Oncol 2003;14(1):91–96.
53. Huddart RA, Norman A, Shahidi M, et al. Cardiovascular disease as a long-term complication of treatment for testicular cancer. J Clin Oncol 2003;21(8):1513–1523.
54. Meinardi MT, Gietema JA, van der Graaf WT, et al. Cardiovascular morbidity in long-term survivors of metastatic testicular cancer. J Clin Oncol 2000;18(8):1725–1732.
55. Travis LB, Andersson M, Gospodarowicz M, et al. Treatment-associated leukemia following testicular cancer. J Natl Cancer Inst 2000;92(14):1165–1171.
56. Bokemeyer C, Berger CC, Kuczyk MA, Schmoll HJ. Evaluation of long-term toxicity after chemotherapy for testicular cancer. J Clin Oncol 1996;14(11):2923–2932.
57. Bokemeyer C, Berger CC, Hartmann JT, et al. Analysis of risk factors for cisplatin-induced ototoxicity in patients with testicular cancer. Br J Cancer 1998;77(8):1355–1362.

10

Surgery for Testicular Cancer

Gillian L. Smith and Timothy J. Christmas

Key Points

1. There is no place for RPLND in the treatment of stage II germ cell tumours or for the staging of stage I disease.
2. RPLND is curative for patients with residual masses post chemotherapy.
3. Surgery for post treatment residual masses should only be carried out in centres of excellence.

Introduction

Testicular germ cell tumors are highly curable, even when metastatic at presentation. Although this is largely because of their sensitivity to platinum-based chemotherapy, well-timed surgical intervention is also crucial in achieving a high cure rate. The diagnosis is usually established by inguinal orchidectomy, and orchidectomy alone represents adequate treatment for many patients. Operative removal of metastatic disease, usually after chemotherapy, is also highly effective and may be curative. Thus the importance of surgical treatment for testicular cancer should not be underestimated.

Inguinal Orchidectomy

Timing of Orchidectomy

Inguinal orchidectomy is the first step in the management and staging of most patients presenting with testicular cancer. Certainly, well patients presenting with a solid testicular mass, the most common presentation, should undergo inguinal orchidectomy as soon as possible followed by radiological staging and referral to an oncologist. In the less common situation of an ill patient with metastases typical of a germ cell tumor and elevated β-human chorionic gonadotropin (βHCG), α-fetoprotein (α-FP), or lactate dehydrogenase (LDH), orchidectomy can be scheduled for after completion of chemotherapy as prognosis may be adversely affected by delaying chemotherapy. Orchidectomy of the affected testis should be performed even if the tumor appears to resolve after chemotherapy, as the testis can be a sanctuary site for persistent active tumor.

Surgical Approach

An inguinal, rather than scrotal, incision should be employed to avoid tumor contamination of the scrotal skin and exposure of the inguinal lymph nodes to the risk of metastasis. In a meta-analysis, scrotal violation increased the risk of local recurrence from 0.4% to 2.9% [1]. The excess risk applied mainly in cases where gross tumor spillage had occurred.

Surgery may be carried out under general or regional anesthesia. A skin crease incision is made over the external inguinal ring, the size depending on the size of the tumor. For a very large tumor, the medial end of the incision can be curved down onto the scrotum allowing resection of a tumor of any size.

The subcutaneous tissues are divided and the external oblique opened to the external ring. A self-retaining retractor aids exposure. The ilioinguinal nerve should be preserved if possible. The cord is mobilized in the inguinal canal. If there is uncertainty about the diagnosis of tumor, a noncrushing bowel clamp or a soft Penrose drain may be used to clamp the cord at this stage. In most cases, however, the preoperative diagnosis of tumor is effectively certain and the cord may be clamped with an artery forceps or ligated at this stage. The cord should be mobilized up to the internal ring, where it should be both ligated and transfixed with nonabsorbable suture material. This ensures clearance of all distal cord structures so that if later retroperitoneal lymph node dissection (RPLND) is required the inguinal canal is already empty and does not require further clearance. The use of a nonabsorbable suture (e.g., Prolene) to transfix or ligate the cut end of the divided cord facilitates identification of the distal end of the cord at RPLND. The testis is then mobilized from the scrotum. Gentle pressure from below and traction on the cord deliver the testis into the incision. The gubernacular attachments can then be divided using the hand-held diathermy spatula with careful attention to hemostasis. Intraoperative local anesthetic infiltration of wound edges and nerves aids postoperative analgesia. Wound lavage with water may be tumoricidal. An inguinal orchidectomy specimen is shown in Figure 10.1.

Complications

Inguinal orchidectomy is generally well tolerated by patients and can be performed as a day case procedure. The most serious complication is scrotal or retroperitoneal hematoma. The risk can be minimized by careful attention to hemostasis and meticulous transfixion and ligation of the divided cord at the internal inguinal ring.

Testicular Prostheses

A testicular prosthesis can be inserted at the time of orchidectomy if the patient wishes. Testicular prostheses were previously manufactured using a solid shell containing a silicon gel core. Concerns were expressed in the early 1990s about such designs in breast prostheses, and a possible association with autoimmune diseases. No causal relationship has been established, although histological and serological evidence of silicone shedding has been identified [2,3]. Currently manufacturers employ either (solid) silicone elastomer or a saline filled silicone shell.

Strict asepsis is essential during insertion and many surgeons administer prophylactic broad-spectrum antibiotics during the procedure. The prosthesis is placed in the scrotum via the inguinal incision. An anchoring suture may be employed, but care should be taken to ensure an appropriate lie and position, and symmetry of size selection. An inguinal approach should be used

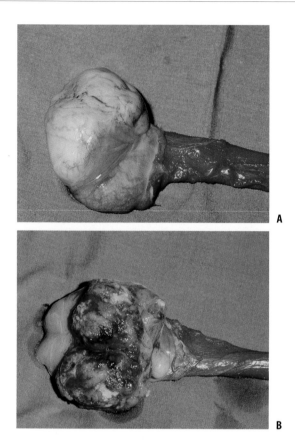

Fig. 10.1. A: Inguinal orchidectomy specimen. B: Inguinal orchidectomy specimen bivalved to demonstrate tumor.

for delayed as well as immediate insertion of a prosthesis, as erosion through scrotal incisions is well recognized.

The most troublesome complication is infection, which often necessitates removal of the prosthesis. In the long term, satisfaction with testicular prostheses is variable. Encapsulation resulting in hardening can occur with time, resulting in a less natural texture. In one series 27% of men were dissatisfied and felt that they had an average or poor cosmetic result [4]. In another series, 20% of patients felt uncomfortable in sexual encounters and only

58% were happy with their sex life [5]. Patients therefore should be counseled appropriately preoperatively and many will opt simply to have an orchidectomy without prosthesis.

Partial Orchidectomy

Partial orchidectomy may be considered in patients with a tumor in a solitary testis or bilateral tumors. The advantage is that it may allow the patient to avoid hormone replacement therapy and, in some cases, to preserve fertility. In a series of 73 men who underwent partial orchidectomy for testicular cancer (primarily seminoma), 85% avoided the need for subsequent hormone replacement. In 82% of patients there was associated carcinoma in situ (CIS) treated with local irradiation (18 Gy). One patient died of systemic tumor progression. There were no local recurrences in the men with CIS who received radiotherapy. There were four local recurrences in patients not irradiated, but all were treated successfully with inguinal orchidectomy. Of 10 men who postponed radiotherapy for fertility reasons, five fathered a child after organ-sparing surgery [6]. The procedure does require specialist expertise, and patients should be referred to a center with experience with partial orchidectomy. Specialist techniques that may be involved are preoperative scrotal magnetic resonance imaging (MRI), intraoperative ultrasound, and frozen section. Intraoperative cooling can be helpful, as Sertoli cells will be morphologically altered after 30 minutes of warm ischemia. Preoperative counseling is vital regarding the potential need for completion orchidectomy, the risk of local recurrence, and the possibility of requiring hormone replacement therapy. Preoperative semen storage should be offered, and patients must be able to comply with intensive follow-up.

Contralateral Testicular Biopsy

Carcinoma in situ (intratubular germ cell neoplasia [ITGCN]) consists of atypical cells located in a single row at the basement membrane of seminiferous tubules. It is universally detected in the tissue surrounding germ cell tumors [7]. These cells are the uniform precursor of all germ cell neoplasms of the testis (other than spermatocytic seminoma) and develop during embryogenesis. Cellular proliferation then probably occurs during and after puberty [8]. Usually all spermatogenic cells are replaced as the CIS cells spread longitudinally along the tubules, leaving only CIS cells and Sertoli cells in a multifocal distribution. Fifty percent of men with ITGCN progress to invasive cancer in 5 years [9,10]. It is unknown whether nonseminomatous tumors develop via a stage of seminoma or progress directly. In view of the high progression rate to invasive tumors, it is desirable to detect CIS by biopsy so that it can be treated before progression occurs.

The following are risk factors for CIS of the residual testis in men with germ cell tumors:

- Age less than 30 years
- Small volume testes (<12 mL)
- Gonadal dysgenesis syndromes
- History of cryptorchid testis (2–3% have CIS)
- Extragonadal germ cell tumor (42% men with primary retroperitoneal disease have CIS)
- Abnormal spermatogenesis (oligozoospermia on semen analysis) (0.4–1.1% of infertile men have CIS)
- Microcalcification (remains controversial)

The potential drawbacks of contralateral testicular biopsy include a 15% to 20% complication rate, with the possibility of impaired hormone production or fertility as a consequence. If CIS is confirmed, radiotherapy does result in irreversible infertility. Most patients who do develop metachronous tumors can be cured with inguinal orchidectomy at the time of recurrence. Thus the potential advantages of preventing second tumors in those with CIS have to be weighed against the possibility of damaging residual testicular function in patients without CIS who have nothing to gain from a biopsy. Most units, therefore, adopt a selective approach to biopsies of the contralateral testis carrying out biopsies in the groups at increased risk. Patients with negative biopsies do require follow-up despite the negative result, as there is a small false-negative rate (0.3%).

Surgical open (stab) biopsy should be undertaken laterally in the upper pole to avoid intratesticular vasculature. The sample should be fixed immediately to preserve architecture ideally in Bouin's solution although formalin suffices. A $3 \times 3 \times 3$ mm biopsy will almost certainly detect CIS if it is present in at least 10% of the tubules. Eighteen-gauge core needle biopsies are probably comparable and take deeper cores [11]. The biopsy may be synchronous with the initial orchidectomy or deferred depending on the clinical scenario.

Retroperitoneal Lymph Node Dissection for Testicular Tumors

Germ Cell Tumors

For a long time it has been recognized that the primary location for the spread of nonseminomatous germ cell of the testis (NSGCT) is the chain of lymph nodes in the retroperitoneum surrounding the aorta and inferior vena cava (IVC). Back in 1897 removal of inguinal lymph nodes at the time radical orchidectomy was recommended [12]. However, when surgeons subsequently became more aware of the lymphatic drainage of the testis, RPLND was advocated and was performed at the same time as radical orchidectomy for testis cancer [13,14]. The location of nodal metastases from the testis was later mapped out in precise detail in men undergoing RPLND for metastatic testis cancer. The most common location for nodal metastases emanating from the right-sided tumors was found to be the aortocaval groove area, whereas left-sided tumors initially spread to the left para-aortic region [15,16]. The RPLND procedure has been a popular treatment for clinical stage II NSGCT and also as a staging procedure (and sometimes of therapeutic benefit) for clinical stage I NSGCT. However, in the modern era the major role for surgery in the treatment of testis cancer has been to establish the diagnosis by radical orchidectomy. Since the advent of platinum-based chemotherapy, many patients with metastatic testis cancer have been cured after orchidectomy by chemotherapy alone. About 25% of men with stage II to IV NSGCT have a residual mass after an intensive course of platinum-based chemotherapy [17]. When the residual mass is greater than 1 to 2 cm in diameter, then postchemotherapy RPLND (PC-RPLND) is indicated as well as excision of residual masses from other sites such as the chest, liver, and brain. When an active tumor recurrence develops after PC-RPLND, further chemotherapy is warranted, and in certain circumstances autologous bone marrow transplantation may be necessary to allow further high-dose chemotherapy. In a few cases further relapse may occur when the disease becomes resistant to chemotherapy, and then "desperation" RPLND (D-RPLND) may be indicated [18].

RPLND for Stage I NSGCT

There has been a trans-Atlantic division of opinion on the role of RPLND for clinical stage I NSGCT. It is usual practice to perform RPLND for clinical stage I NSGCT in some centers in the United States [19]. The rationale behind this is that approximately 30% to 35% of clinical stage I patients are in fact pathological stage II [20]. In men with tumor within the nodes, up to 60% may be cured by RPLND alone, and those who do relapse do so away from the retroperitoneum. Furthermore, because the sympathetic nerve fibers that subserve ejaculation are now identifiable and the anatomy well recognized [21], it is possible to perform nerve-sparing RPLND in men with such low-volume lymph nodes, hence preserving ejaculation. The alternatives to RPLND for stage I disease are long-term surveillance or adjuvant chemotherapy. Chemotherapy would normally be considered only in high risk patients with malignant teratoma undifferentiated (MTU) in the primary tumor and vascular invasion within the testis/cord. Surveillance is the most popular option in most countries; in a survey of 273 urologists in the United Kingdom all patients with clinical stage I NSGCT were referred to major cancer centers for surveillance [22]. Comparison between surveillance and RPLND for stage I disease reveals similar mortality figures. However, it has been argued that primary RPLND is more likely to preserve fertility because fewer patients require chemotherapy, and retroperitoneal relapse in the surveillance group may also necessitate PC-RPLND, which may compromise ejaculation if the sympathetic nerves cannot be preserved [23].

RPLND for Stage II NSGCT

Since the advent of the platinum-based chemotherapy era, most men with clinical stage II NSGCT are treated with chemotherapy. However, the Indiana University group has advocated primary RPLND for stage II NSGCT and has compared the results with similar patients treated with platinum-based chemotherapy. Both treatments were curative as monotherapy in 67%; survival was

98% in those treated by RPLND and 96% who had primary chemotherapy. Late relapse and toxicity rates were greater in the chemotherapy group [24,25]. However, in spite of the findings in Indianapolis, the favored primary treatment for stage II testicular NSGCT is chemotherapy.

Postchemotherapy RPLND

After an intensive course of platinum-based chemotherapy for stage II to IV NSGCT of the testis, a residual mass will be apparent within the retroperitoneum on computed tomography (CT) or MRI scans (Fig. 10.2) in 25% or more cases [26]. It is now established practice to excise such residual masses in order to increase the chance of cure [27]. However, when the mass is <1 cm in diameter, it most likely contains necrotic tissue only [28] and can be safely observed [29]. Patients with malignant teratoma intermediate that contains differentiated teratoma (MTI) are at risk of the tumor masses becoming cystic and enlarging during chemotherapy. Enlarging masses with falling tumor markers are characteristic of "growing teratoma syndrome," which requires surgical removal of all tumor masses. All patients with MTI should have a CT scan after two or three courses of chemotherapy as masses in "growing teratoma syndrome" can become inoperable and

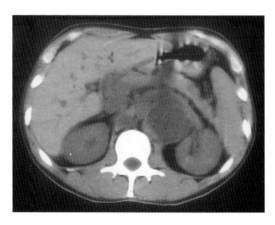

Fig. 10.2. Computed tomography (CT) scan showing residual retroperitoneal nodal mass after chemotherapy for stage II germ cell tumor of the testis.

there may be only a limited window of opportunity in which to plan successful surgery. Patients who relapse after an initial response to chemotherapy should always be worked up to locate any tumor masses that might be resectable. Development of new masses, enlargement of previously known masses, or positivity on positron emission tomography (PET) scan can indicate the masses most likely to contain active tumor. Resection of all apparent disease with subsequent fall of tumor markers to normal can avoid further chemotherapy in a proportion of patients.

The objective of PC-RPLND in men with residual masses is to excise all the remaining tissue. Incomplete excision is associated with a considerably worse prognosis [27]. After PC-RPLND, decision making regarding follow-up and further therapy depends on the result of histological examination of the resected tissue. In the authors' personal series of 303 cases of PC-RPLND for NSGCT performed between 1993 and 2004, the overall survival rate is over 90%. This series includes a number of patients who had recurred after previous PC-RPLND performed at other hospitals; this has been shown to worsen the long-term chance of survival [30]. Approximately half of the resected specimens contained differentiated teratoma (TD); just over one fifth contained necrosis/fibrosis only; and the remainder contained active malignancy (MTU, yolk sac tumor, choriocarcinoma, sarcoma, neuroectodermal tumor, or carcinoma). These findings are similar to those of other large series of PC-RPLND [27]. Factors that increase the chance of finding active tumor in the resected specimen are persistent elevation of tumor markers, large size, failure to serially decrease in size, and history of relapse. Factors that increase the chance of finding differentiated teratoma are presence of MTI initially and heterogeneous or cystic masses on CT scans.

Nearly all patients with necrosis/fibrosis in the specimen are cured but should be followed up in the long-term (Fig. 10.3). Those men with TD in the specimen have a >95% chance of cure, provided that all residual tissue has been removed. Malignant tissue within the PC-RPLND specimen confers a worse prognosis. The majority of these patients are best treated with further chemotherapy, sometimes a high-dose regimen including Taxol with autologous bone marrow transplantation. When a further recurrence occurs after a second course of chemotherapy, then desperation RPLND can be considered and is likely to be of benefit in up to 50% [31]. All men who have undergone PC-

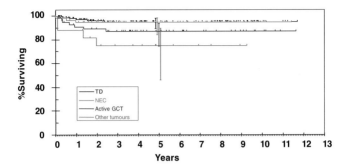

Fig. 10.3. Cause specific survival after postchemotherapy retroperitoneal lymph node dissection (RPLND) for nonseminomatous germ cell of the testis (NSGCT) of the testis according to histology of the resected specimen. TD, differentiated teratoma; NEC, necrosis; GCT, germ cell tumors.

RPLND should remain under follow-up because there is a 2% risk of developing a contralateral tumor, and recurrence can occur beyond 15 years after PC-RPLND [32].

Seminoma

Patients with seminoma may have residual masses following chemotherapy. These masses are often associated with a fibrous reaction that makes retroperitoneal surgery more difficult. In the majority of cases, these masses are best observed due to the difficulty of removing them and the high chance that they will not contain active tumor. Patients with a seminomatous element in their germ cell tumors do have a higher rate of intra- and postoperative complications than patients with pure NSGCT undergoing postchemotherapy RPLND. Additional procedures such as nephrectomy and vascular interventions are more commonly required [33].

Stromal Tumors

Stromal tumors of the testis (e.g., Leydig, Sertoli, and granulosa cell tumors) are uncommon, accounting for about 2% of adult testicular tumors. Most do not behave in a malignant fashion and can be cured by orchidectomy, but approximately 10% have metastatic potential. In contrast with treatment for germ cell tumors, treatment for metastatic stromal tumors is not very effective. Patients with a malignant stromal tumor that metastasizes survive on average only 3 years from diagnosis. In addition, it is difficult to identify high-risk patients who might benefit from more intensive treatment or surveillance, as there are no consistently reliable histolog-ical indicators of malignant potential. Although several adverse features have been described, accurate prediction of aggressive tumor behavior in individual cases remains difficult. Experience with these tumors and the potential for clinical trials are limited by the small numbers of patients and there is therefore no consensus on the best treatment. A number of studies have suggested that there is a role for prophylactic RPLND in stage I stromal tumors [34–36]. Early results suggest that the procedure is safe in this group of patients, although the long-term effect on survival is not yet known.

Surgical Technique

In all stage I cases it is possible to perform RPLND through a midline abdominal incision, and the same applies to men undergoing low volume PC-RPLND. A thoracoabdominal approach (Fig. 10.4) affords excellent exposure for resection of large-volume disease. The thoracoabdominal incision is also advanta-

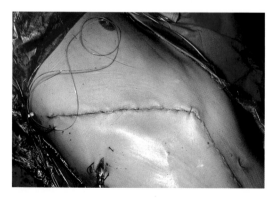

Fig. 10.4. Thoracoabdominal incision for postchemotherapy RPLND.

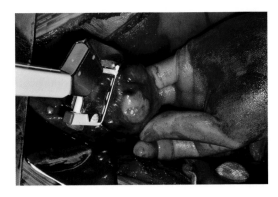

Fig. 10.5. Resection of a small lung metastasis using a stapling device at thoracoab-dominal postchemotherapy RPLND.

geous when there is residual disease within both the retro-peritoneum and thoracic cavity, as it allows synchronous excision of pulmonary metastases (Fig. 10.5) [37] and intrathoracic lymph nodes [38].

Complete bilateral RPLND has in the past been shown to lead to loss of ejaculation due to excision of sympathetic nerve fibers surrounding the aorta and IVC [39]. We now know much more about the distribution of nodal metastases from testis cancer [16] and the anatomy of the sympathetic nerves [21], which together have resulted in the development of modified templates for RPLND. In the case of left-sided tumors, a template nodal excision is performed in an area bounded by the left renal vein, aorta, left common iliac artery, and the left ureter. The midaorta, right common iliac artery, right ureter, and right renal vein bound the right-sided template. Although it may not be possible to preserve all sympathetic nerve fibers during RPLND, the use of a modified template should reduce damage to contralateral sympathetic fibers and hence prevent anejaculation after surgery [40].

The objective in PC-RPLND is to remove all the residual mass, and this may also necessitate excision of adjacent structures such as the kidney [41], the aorta, and the IVC [42]. Hence, it advisable that the surgeon performing RPLND be able to undertake such procedures or call for assistance from another surgeon at short notice.

Complications

The operative mortality of RPLND is low at less than 1% [43]. In one large series of primary nerve sparing RPLND for stage I NSGCT, only 5.4% of patients developed complications that prolonged hospital stay by more than 2 days. Antegrade ejaculation was preserved in most patients (93.3%) [44]. The postoperative complication rate of postchemotherapy RPLND is reported as around 7%, with most patients tolerating surgery well and recovering uneventfully [45]. Postchemotherapy patients may have diminished pulmonary, renal, and nutritional reserves, and are more likely to have a large disease burden necessitating longer and more extensive surgery with a higher risk of additional procedures such as nephrectomy, bowel resection, and vascular repair. The most common perioperative complications are wound infection and prolonged ileus. Acute renal failure, pancreatitis, ascites, and pulmonary complications are also recognized. Ejaculatory dysfunction is the main long-term complication.

Conclusion

The ability to cure the great majority of men with testis cancer has generally been attributed to platinum-based chemotherapy. However, the role of RPLND should not be underestimated. In low-stage NSGCT, surveillance (stage I) and primary chemotherapy (stage II) have in most centers replaced primary RPLND, and PC-RPLND is a crucial adjunct to chemotherapy, enabling a very high cure rate for more advanced stages of NSGCT. The best chance of cure is when complete excision of the residual masses after chemotherapy is achieved, and this is most likely to be the case in a specialized cancer center [27,30].

Controversies and Outstanding Issues

1. There are no major controversies?
2. Efforts need to be made to continue the trend to centralise surgery.

References

1. Capelouto CC, Clark PE, Ransil BJ, Loughlin KR. A review of scrotal violation in testicular cancer: is adjuvant local therapy necessary? J Urol 1995;153:981–985.
2. Barrett DM, O'Sullivan DC, Malizia AA, et al. Particle shedding and migration from silicone genitourinary prosthetic devices. J Urol 1991;146:319–322.
3. Henderson J, Culkin D, Mata J, Wilson M, Venable D. Analysis of immunological alterations associated with testicular prostheses. J Urol 1995;154:1748–1751.
4. Adshead J, Khoubehi B, Wood J, Rustin G. Testicular implants and patient satisfaction: a questionnaire-based study of men after orchidectomy for testicular cancer. BJU Int 2001;88(6):559–562.
5. Incrocci L, Bosch JL, Slob AK. Testicular prostheses: body image and sexual functioning. BJU Int 1999;84(9):1043–1045.
6. Heidenreich A, Albers P, Hartmann M, Kliesch S, Kohrmann KU, Dleckmann KP, German Testicular Cancer Study Group. Organ sparing surgery for malignant germ cell tumor of the testis. J Urol 2001;166:2161–2165.
7. Skakkebaek NE. Possible carcinoma-in-situ of testis. Lancet 1992;2(7776):516–517.
8. Skakkebaek NE, Rajpert-De Meyts E, Jorgensen N, et al. Germ cell cancer and disorders of spermatogenesis: an environmental connection? Acta Pathol Microbial Scand 1998;106:3–11.
9. Bettocchi C, Coker CB, Deacon J, Parkinson C, Pryor JP. A review of testicular intratubular germ cell neoplasia in infertile men. J Androl 1994;15(suppl):14S–16S.
10. Montironi R. Intratubular germ cell neoplasia of the testis: testicular intraepithelial neoplasia. Eur Urol 2002;41:651–654.
11. Harland S, Cook PA, Fossa SD, et al. Intratubular germ cell neoplasia of the contralateral testis in testicular cancer: defining a high risk group. J Urol 1998;16:1353–1357.
12. Stimson JC. A new operation for malignant tumors of the testicle. The necessity of a more extensive operation than castration for carcinoma, sarcoma of the testicle. Medical Record 1897;52:623.
13. Roberts JB. Excision of the lumbar lymph nodes and spermatic vein in malignant tumors of the testicle. Am J Surg 1902;36:539.
14. Bland-Sutton J. An operation for lumbar gland removal in cases of testis tumour. Lancet 1909;1:1406.
15. Ray B, Hajdu SI, Whitmore WF. Distribution of retroperitoneal lymph node metastases in testicular germinal tumors. Cancer 1973; 33:340–348.
16. Donohue JP, Zachary JM, Maynard BR. Distribution of nodal metastases in nonseminomatous testis cancer. J Urol 1982;128:315–320.

17. Hendry WF. Decision making in abdominal surgery following chemotherapy for testicular cancer. Eur J Cancer 1995;5:649–650.

18. Nichols CR, Saxman S. Primary salvage treatment of recurrent germ cell tumors: experience at Indiana University. Semin Oncol 1998;25:210–214.

19. Donohue JP, Thornhill JA, Foster RS, et al. Retroperitoneal lymphadenectomy for clinical stage A testis cancer (1965 to 1989): modifications of technique and impact on ejaculation. J Urol 1993;149:237–243.

20. Foster RS, Donohue JP. Surgical treatment of clinical stage A non-seminomatous testis cancer. Semin Oncol 1992;19:166–170.

21. Foster RS, Donohue JP. Nerve-sparing retroperitoneal lymphadenectomy. Urol Clin North Am 1993;20:117–125.

22. Bower M, Ma R, Savage P, et al. British urological surgery practice: 2. Renal, bladder and testis cancer. Br J Urol 1998;81:513–517.

23. Foster RS, McNulty A, Rubin LR, et al. The fertility of patients with clinical stage I testis cancer managed by nerve sparing retroperitoneal lymph node dissection [see comments]. J Urol 1994;152:1139–1142.

24. Donohue JP, Thornhill JA, Foster RS, et al. The role of retroperitoneal lymphadenectomy in clinical stage B testis cancer: the Indiana University experience (1965 to 1989). J Urol 1995;153:85–89.

25. Baniel J, Sella A. Complications of retroperitoneal lymph node dissection in testicular cancer: primary and post-chemotherapy. Semin Surg Oncol 1999;17(4):263–267.

26. Tait D, Peckham MJ, Hendry WF, Goldstraw P. Post-chemotherapy surgery in advanced non-seminomatous germ cell testicular tumours: the significance of histology with particular reference to differentiated (mature) teratoma. Br J Cancer 1984;50:601–609.

27. Hendry WF, A'Hern RP, Hetherington JW, et al. Para-aortic lymphadenectomy after chemotherapy for metastatic non-seminomatous germ cell tumours: prognostic value and therapeutic benefit. Br J Urol 1993;71:208–213.

28. Janetschek G, Hobisch A, Hittmair A, et al. Laparoscopic retroperitoneal lymphadenectomy after chemotherapy for stage IIB non-seminomatous testicular carcinoma. J Urol 1999;161:477–481.

29. Napier MP, Naraghi A, Christmas TJ, Rustin GJ. Long-term follow-up of residual masses after chemotherapy in patients with non-seminomatous germ cell tumours. Br J Cancer 2000;83:1274–1280.

30. Christmas TJ, Smith GL, Kooner RS. Reoperation for metastatic testis cancer after chemotherapy. J Urol 1998;159(suppl):49.

31. Ravi R, Ong J, Oiver RT, et al. Surgery as salvage therapy in chemotherapy-resistant nonseminomatous germ cell tumours. Br J Urol 1998;81:884–888.

32. Elkabir JJ, Christmas TJ, Ellamushi H, Mendoza N. Late relapse of metastatic teratoma invading a vertebral body: a combined surgical approach. Br J Urol 1997;79:999–1000.

33. Mosharafa AA, Foster RS, Leibovich BC, Bihrle R, Johnson C, Donohue JP. Is post-chemotherapy resection of seminomatous elements associated with higher acute morbidity? J Urol 2003;169: 2126–2128.

34. Mosharafa AA, Foster RS, Bihrle R, et al. Does retroperitoneal lymph node dissection have a curative role for patients with sex cord-stromal testicular tumors? Cancer 2003;98(4):753–757.

35. Smith GL, Christmas TJ, Seckl MJ, Rustin GJS. The role of retroperitoneal lymph node dissection in the management of stromal tumours of the testis. BJU Int 2003;91(suppl):61.

36. Peschel R, Gettman MT, Steiner H, Neururer R, Bartsch G. Management of adult Leydig-cell testicular tumors: assessing the role of laparoscopic retroperitoneal lymph node dissection. J Endourol 2003;17:777–780.

37. Christmas TJ, Smith GL, Kooner RS. Wedge resection of pulmonary metastases from cancer of the testis or kidney using a vascular staple device. Br J Urol 1998;81(6):911–912.

38. Christmas TJ, Doherty AP, Bower M. Retrocrural lymph node metastases from testis germ cell tumours: removal via a thoracoabdominal extraperitoneal approach after chemotherapy. Br J Urol 1997;79(3):468–470.

39. Leiter E, Brendler H. Loss of ejaculation following bilateral retroperitoneal lymphadenectomy. J Urol 1967;98:375–378.

40. Donohue JP, Foster RS, Rowland RG, et al. Nerve-sparing retroperitoneal lymphadenectomy with preservation of ejaculation. J Urol 1990;144:287–291.

41. Nash PA, Leibovitch I, Foster RS, et al. En bloc nephrectomy in patients undergoing post-chemotherapy retroperitoneal lymph node dissection for nonseminomatous testis cancer: indications, implications and outcomes. J Urol 1998;159:707–710.

42. Christmas TJ, Smith GL, Kooner R. Vascular interventions during post-chemotherapy retroperitoneal lymph-node dissection for metastatic testis cancer. Eur J Surg Oncol 1998;24(4):292–297.

43. Baniel J, Foster RS, Rowland RG, et al. Complications of post-chemotherapy retroperitoneal lymph node dissection. J Urol 1995; 153:976–980.

44. Heidenreich, A, Albers P, Hartmann M, et al., German Testicular Cancer Study Group. Complications of primary nerve sparing retroperitoneal lymph node dissection for clinical stage I nonseminomatous germ cell tumors of the testis: experience of the German Testicular Cancer Study Group. J Urol 2003;169:1710–1714.

45. Mosharafa AA, Foster RS, Koch MO, Bihrle R, Donohue JP. Complications of post-chemotherapy retroperitoneal lymph node dissection for testis cancer. J Urol 2004;171:1839–1841.
46. Christmas TJ, Doherty AP, Rustin HJ, et al. Excision of residual masses of metastatic germ cell tumours after chemotherapy: the role of extra-peritoneal surgical approaches. Br J Urol 1998;81:301–308.

11

The Clinical Management of Penile Cancer

Rajiv Sarin, Hemant B. Tongaonkar, and Reena Engineer

Key Points

1. Preservation of organ function is clearly important.
2. Optimal radiotherapy is effective in early localised tumours
2. Surgery is the mainstay of treatment for advanced local disease and involved groin nodes.
3. There is no role for prophylactic lymphadenectomy.
4. For advanced inoperable cancers concurrent chemoradiotherapy is appropriate.

Epidemiology and Etiology

Penile malignancies are uncommon in most parts of the world, but there is a striking geographical variation around the world. While the age-adjusted incidence rate is less than 1 per 100,000 in Europe and North America, in parts of South America, Africa, and India, the incidence is as high as 12 per 100,000 men [1]. Even within a country, there are marked regional variations. In Brazil the incidence of penile cancer is as high as 28 and 50 per 100,000 men in the cities of Sao Paulo and Recife, respectively [2]. Within Africa, the highest incidence has been reported from Uganda, where it is the most common cancer in males [3]. In India the disease is more common in the rural population with an incidence of 3 per 100,000 people accounting for more than 6% of all cancers in rural men [4].

In a review of risk factors for the development of penile cancers, strong risk factors identified with an odds ratio of more than 10 were phimosis, chronic inflammatory conditions such as balanoposthitis, lichen sclerosis et atrophicus, and treatment with psoralen and ultraviolet A [5]. A three- to fivefold increased risk was found for smoking, sexual history, and condyloma. Circumcision in the neonatal period was associated with a threefold decreased risk of penile cancer. Human papillomavirus (HPV) DNA has been identified in 40% to 50% of invasive penile carcinoma and 70% to 100% of carcinoma in situ [5].

Natural History, Histology, and Clinical Presentation

Penile cancers are diagnosed often in the fifth to seventh decade in the West [3], but in high incidence areas, the disease often manifests one to two decade earlier [2,6,7]. The disease starts from the glans, corona, or prepuce, but in certain parts of the world where delayed presentation is common, the majority of patients have tumor extension to penile shaft or groin nodes at the time of diagnosis [7]. A vast majority of these invasive cancers are squamous carcinomas or their variants such as verrucous or basaloid carcinoma, and other histologies are very rare [3]. The natural history of penile in situ carcinoma has not been studied as extensively as cervical intraepithelial neoplasia. Some reports suggest more aggressive behavior for in situ penile carcinoma with recurrence within 5 years in most cases, with carcinoma in situ at the resection margin [8]. Carcinoma in situ or dysplasia has been reported in one fourth of patients with invasive penile carcinoma [9]. Certain premalignant lesions of the penis have been identified, which may progress to invasive penile cancer over a variable length of time (e.g., leukoplakia, erythroplasia of Queyrat, Bowen's disease, Buschke-Löwenstein tumor, balanitis xerotica obliterans, etc.). The nomenclature of precancerous lesions in this fashion is quite confusing and the use of terms *penile intra-epithelial neoplasia grade I, II, III* or *squamous intraepithelial lesions of low and high grade* are recommended to avoid such confusion [10].

Local Spread

Penile carcinomas arise from the mucosa of the glans or coronal sulcus and sometimes from the foreskin of uncircumcised men. The clinical manifestation depends on the histological type of the tumor and any time lag before the diagnosis. The initial lesion may be warty or verrucous, ulcerative, proliferative, ulceroproliferative, or sometimes like a plaque over the glans. The tumor then invades deeply to involve the corpus cavernosa and spongiosum, urethra, and skin of the shaft, and in very advanced cases it involves the perineum, scrotum, or prostate.

One of the most elegant studies of clinicopathological correlation in penile carcinoma was reported by Cubilla et al. [11] in 1993. On the basis of a detailed examination of whole organ sections of 66 penile resections, they described the following clinicopathological variants: (a) *verrucous carcinoma* (18%): these papillary exophytic tumors of low histological grade are locally aggressive but vascular or perineural invasion and lymph node metastases are rare; (b) *superficially spreading carcinoma* (42%): this commonest variety presented with centrifugal or radial growth to large areas of the epithelial compartments such as the glans, coronal sulcus, and the foreskin; (c) *vertical growth carcinoma* (32%): these unifocal tumors are characteristically aggressive, infiltrating deep anatomical structures, and have a higher histological grade and a higher propensity for lymph node metastases; and (d) *multicentric carcinoma* (8%): an uncommon variety in which there is normal epithelium in between the multiple foci of carcinoma. The pattern of spread of the superficially spreading carcinoma and multicentric carcinomas suggests that glans mucosa, coronal sulcus, and foreskin may be considered as a single field susceptible to malignant transformation.

Nodal Metastasis

Like all squamous carcinomas, penile cancers have a propensity for lymphatic spread to the draining lymph nodes in the superficial and deep inguinal region and later to the iliac chain. Skip metastasis to the iliac nodes is very unusual [12,13]. Lymphatic spread is uncommon in the verrucous cancers of the penis [9,11]. For invasive squamous carcinomas, the risk of nodal metastases increases with increasing depth of invasion [12–14],

Table 11.1. Incidence of nodal metastasis for different T stage and histological grades of penile carcinoma

Author [reference]	Nodal metastasis (%) in patients with T1, well or moderately well differentiated tumors	Nodal metastasis (%) in patients with corporal invasion
Solsona et al. [13]	1/17 (6%)	27/42 (64%)
Fraley et al. [16]	1/19 (5%)	26/29 (90%)
Theodorescu et al. [17]	2/18 (11%)	12/18 (67%)
Heyns et al. [18]	5/91 (5%)	15/32 (47%)
Total	9/145 (6%)	80/121 (66%)

higher T stage, and histological grade [12,15]. Early cancers without corporal invasion and low or intermediate histological grade have a 6% incidence of nodal metastasis as opposed to 66% risk in tumors with corporal invasion or high grade as shown in Table 11.1. Solsona et al. [13] identified three risk categories for nodal metastases. The frequency of nodal metastasis in low risk (T1 G1) was 0/19; intermediate risk (T1 G2/3 or T2/3 G1) was 8/22 (36%); and high risk (T2/3 G3) was 20/25 (80%). However, tumor infiltration of the corpora cavernosa, urethra, and adjacent structures was not confirmed as a predictor of nodal metastasis in a multivariate analysis of 145 Brazilians [19]. Venous and lymphatic embolization was the only significant predictor of lymph node metastasis in this study.

Metastatic spread to bones, lung, or other organs at presentation is rare. However, during follow up, 5% to 10% of patients may develop distant metastases, generally in the setting of uncontrolled locoregional disease [3].

Pretreatment Evaluation and Pitfalls in Staging

For optimum management using the most appropriate treatment approach and ensuring best outcome, a simple but systematic pretreatment evaluation is mandatory. A careful history and interview should also include a history of sexual practices, sexually transmitted disease, chronic inflammatory penile conditions, and the likely psychosexual impact of a penectomy if recommended. The location, type, size, and extension of the tumor, presence of any premalignant or inflammatory condition, infection, or phimosis should be documented after examination by a clinician familiar with this disease. Clinical evaluation of the primary tumor may not detect subclinical infiltration in 10% of cases, whereas in 16% of patients tumor edema and infection may be mistaken for infiltration [20]. In small penile tumors, ultrasound was not found accurate enough in distinguishing invasion of subepithelial connective tissue and invasion into the corpus spongiosum [21]. However, in more advanced tumors, ultrasound was found to be more accurate than clinical examination in estimating the extent of penile tumor, thereby allowing preservation of a longer penile stump during partial penectomy [22]. Magnetic resonance imaging (MRI) with its multiplanar imaging and sharp contrast between different penile structures can identify corporal involvement and local extension with more than 80% accuracy [23].

Evaluation of groin nodes is best done by careful palpation of the groin, fine needle aspiration cytology (FNAC) from any palpable nodes, and computed tomography (CT) scan in cases of clinically suspicious nodes or very obese individuals. Clinical examination of the groin may be fallacious, especially in patient populations that frequently have reactive groin nodes due to chronic infections or those with infected fungating tumors. Palpable nodes may be pathologically negative in 60% cases if the clinical node size is <2 cm and in 10% cases if they measure ≥2 cm [12]. In contrast 15% to 20% of patients with clinically negative groin have unsuspected pathological nodal metastases on groin dissection [24]. In a study comparing various methods for evaluation of nodal metastasis, FNAC, CT scan, and lymphangiography all showed 100% specificity but sensitivity was best for FNAC (71%) as opposed to 36% for CT and 31% for lymphangiography [20].

The first widely used staging systems for penile carcinoma was proposed by Jackson [25] in 1966. After the Union Internationale Contre le Cancer (UICC) tumor, node, metastasis (TNM) staging was published in 1978 and subsequently revised in 1987 [26], Jackson's staging system is now going out of favor. Of the three staging systems shown in Table 11.2, the Jackson and UICC 1978

Table 11.2. Different staging systems for carcinoma penis

Jackson staging, 1966 [25]

Stage 1: Limited to glans and or prepuce
Stage 2: Extending into the shaft or corpora but without nodal
metastases
Stage 3: Confined to the shaft with malignant but operable inguinal
nodes
Stage 4: Invasion beyond shaft, inoperable regional nodes or distant
metastases

UICC TNM staging, 1978 [26]

T stage	N stage
T1: Tumor <2 cm, superficial or exophytic	N0: No nodal involvement
T2: Tumor 2–5 cm or minimal extension	N1: Movable unilateral regional nodes
T3: Tumor >5 cm with deep extension or involvement extensionof urethra	N2: Movable bilateral regional nodes
T4: Infiltrates neighboring structures	N3: Fixed regional lymph nodes

UICC TNM staging, 1987 [26] (not changed in the UICC TNM 1997
version and AJCC TNM 2002 version)

T stage	N stage
T1: Subepithelial connective tissue	N0: No nodal involvement
T2: Corpus spongiosum or cavernosum	N1: One superficial inguinal node
T3: Urethra, prostate	N2: Multiple or bilateral superficial inguinal nodes
T4: Other adjacent structures	N3: Deep inguinal or pelvic nodes

staging is based on clinical examination, whereas the UICC 1987 system is essentially a pathological system. The Jackson staging is based on the involvement of the penile shaft or adjacent structures and the operability of groin nodes. These findings are not only clinically distinguishable but also useful for treatment decision making. However, the main disadvantage of this system is that it groups together tumors with different sizes and different extents of infiltration without considering their prognostic and therapeutic implication. It is also ambiguous about primary tumors confined to the glans but with nodal involvement. In the UICC 1978 system, the T stage is based on tumor size and extent of infiltration and the N stage is based on the laterality and mobility of regional nodes. In the latest revision in the UICC TNM staging of 1987, which has been retained in the 2002 version, the T stage is based on the invasion of the corpus cavernosa and spongiosum, and the N stage is based on the number, laterality, and site (inguinal or iliac) of nodal involvement. Although this provides more refined prognos-tic information, it is essentially a pathological staging system and not suitable for patients who do not undergo a penectomy. Similarly, although it makes a prognostically very important distinction between inguinal and iliac nodal involvement, it has discarded the previous criteria of node operability, a very important determinant of survival. With inherent limitations of each of the three staging systems, the UICC 1978 system is perhaps most appropriate for the initial staging of all cases and as the only staging of patients not undergoing penectomy or groin dissection. The UICC 1987 version is useful as a pathological staging system for patients who undergo penectomy and ilioinguinal node dissection. Replacing the clinical staging system by a pathology-based staging by the UICC has been criticized by most authorities [26].

Biopsy

Histological confirmation of malignancy is mandatory before planning definitive treatment. Patients with small lesions restricted to the prepuce or the penile skin may undergo wide excision of the same with a healthy margin all around, which will be both diagnostic and therapeutic in some cases. Lesions involving the glans, however, require a deep punch or incision biopsy to confirm malignancy and its histological subtype, grade, and invasiveness. In case of a phimotic preputial sac, a dorsal slit or circumcision may be required to obtain an adequate biopsy sample.

Treatment Options, Techniques, and Outcome

With a variety of available treatment options for various stages of the disease, there is no evidence-based consensus regarding the best ther-apeutic approach, especially for early cancers. Although the relative rarity of the disease in the developed countries where most randomized trials are conducted is partly responsible, an equally important reason for the lack of evidence-based consensus is the strong bias among specialists treating this disease. A national survey in the United Kingdom revealed that irrespective of the extent of cancer, the majority of urologists preferred penectomy, whereas clinical oncologists preferred radiotherapy [27].

The management of the primary tumor and nodes has to be considered separately, as the treatment of the primary is always therapeutic but treatment of the nodes may be either prophylactic or therapeutic, sometimes using different treatment modalities for the primary and nodes.

Management of the Penile Primary Tumor

The management of penile primary tumor has gradually evolved in the form of surgery, radiotherapy, and laser excision/ablation. The treatment modality best suited for a patient depends on the patient's age, the size and extension of the tumor, the probability of cure and salvage, and the expected psychosocial impact of amputative surgery. In the absence of any randomized trial or even large comprehensive prospective single-arm studies, and considering the known strong bias for their own specialty among urologists and radiation oncologists [27], one has to exercise great caution in interpreting the avail-able literature. The treatment approach can be broadly categorized as penile conservative therapy (PCT) or penile amputation.

Penile Conservative Therapy

Because amputative surgery for penile cancer may lead to major psychosexual dysfunction, various attempts have been made to devise conservative treatment modalities based on careful oncological, anatomical, and technical considerations. Judicious use of conventional or micrographic surgery, laser ablation, or radiotherapy can allow preservation of a functioning phallus in appropriately selected patients with early cancers. However, there are no comparative studies and no consensus regarding the best modality for PCT. The type of cases suitable for a particular PCT modality depends on the size, site, extent of the tumor, and presence or absence of invasive carcinoma. Circumcision has been reported mostly for cancers limited to the prepuce, conventional/micrographic wide excision for very small superficial invasive carcinoma, laser excision/ablation for in situ or very select superficial invasive carcinoma, and radiotherapy for all variants of early penile cancer. In contrast to 97% to 100% local control rates with partial penectomy for early penile cancer, penile control rate with all these PCT modalities is in the range of 80% to 90% even in appropriately selected cases. Fortunately, almost all penile failures after PCT can be successfully salvaged with a penectomy, thereby allowing preservation of the phallus and better sexual functioning in the vast majority of patients, as shown in Table 11.3.

Wide Excision

For small noninvasive or minimally invasive lesions confined to the prepuce, circumcision may be adequate. Wide excision, with confirmation of an adequate free resection margin by intraoperative frozen section examination, is recommended for small noninvasive or minimally invasive lesions away from the urethra. Strict case selection is imperative because an improper selection of patients for conservative procedures may lead to high local recurrence rates [33–36]. Although Horenblas et al. [37] have reported local recurrence in only two of the 11 patients after wide excision or circumcision, excessive local recurrence rates of 56% for T1 and 100% for T2 tumors was seen after organ-preserving surgical procedures in another study from Heidelberg [38]. Conservative treatments warrant cautious evaluation because of the relatively small number of treated patients and the lack of

Table 11.3. Treatment results of major radiotherapy studies

Author [reference] institute, mean follow-up in years, study period	Treatment modality, median radiation dose (number of patients)	Initial local control	Eventual local control after salvage	Penectomy for necrosis	Urethral stricture rate
Rozan et al. [28], French multicenter, 11.7 years, 1959–1989	Implant alone, 63 Gy (184 patients) Implant, 50 Gy + surgery or external radiotherapy (RT), 40 Gy (75 patients)	218/259 (84%)	16/259 (6%)	19/259 (7%)	79/259 (31%)
Delannes et al. [29], Toulouse, France, 6.9 years, 1971–1989	Implants, 60 Gy (51 patients)	42/51 (82%)	48/51 (94%)	8/51 (16%)	21/51 (41%)
Ravi et al. [30], Cancer Institute, Adyar, India, 11.6 years, 1959–1988	EBRT, 50 to 60 Gy (128 patients) Implants/molds, 60 to 70 Gy (28 patients)	101/156 (65%)	152/156 (97%)	10/156 (6%)	37/156 (24%)

Sarin et al. [31] Royal Marsden, UK, 5.2 years, 1960–1990	EBRT, 60 Gy (56 patients) Implants, 60 Gy (13 patients)	39/69 (57%)	62/69 (90%)	2/69 (3%)	10/69 (14%)
Chaudhary et al. [32], Tata Memorial, India, 2 years, 1988–1996	Implant, 50 Gy	18/23 (78%)	22/23 (96%)	Nil	2/23 (9%)
Present study [unpublished], Tata Memorial, India, 2.5 years, 1996–2003	Accelerated EBRT, 54 to 55 Gy in 16–18 fractions	18/23 (78%)	23/23 (100%)	Nil	Nil

EBRT, external beam radiotherapy.

good-quality comparative data. Besides, the functional and aesthetic results are not always excellent.

Mohs' Micrographic Surgery

This special surgical technique allows for preservation of maximum normal penile tissue and gives results comparable to more radical procedures in patients with small lesions involving distal portion of the glans [38,39]. It entails removal of diseased tissue in thin layers, accurate construction and mapping of excised tissue, and confirmation of negative margins by frozen-section examination of horizontal tissue sections, and it has the capacity to trace out deeper unsuspected extension of the disease. However, when employed for larger lesions, it is rather time-consuming besides resulting in a misshapen glans or meatal stenosis, with an occasional need of correction or reconstruction of the same. Strict case selection is crucial as Mohs reported a 100% local control rate for lesions less than 1 cm but only a 50% local control rate for lesions larger than 3 cm in size.

Laser Therapy

There are many reports of laser therapy, using carbon dioxide and/or neodymium:yttrium-aluminum-garnet (Nd:YAG) lasers for in situ and early invasive penile cancer. In appropriately selected cases laser therapy has the potential for preservation of normal penile tissue and function and local control rates comparable with more radical procedures. Bandiermonte et al. [40] reported CO_2 laser treatment of patients with T1 lesions, with a 15% relapse rate. Subsequently, the Nd:YAG alone or in combination with CO_2 laser has been successfully used either for complete destruction of the lesion or for laser coagulation of the base after partial excision of the tumor, resulting in satisfactory cosmetic results as well as good local control [37,41–44]. Following laser photocoagulation of the tumor base, healing by secondary intention is usually completed by 8 weeks [37]. However, laser therapy has the disadvantages of having uncontrolled depth of excision, not providing adequate tissue for pathological examination, and entailing the need for close follow-up to identify local relapse. Laser therapy is appropriate initial treatment for carcinoma in situ of the penis and select cases of recurrent carcinoma in situ. However, these patients need to be carefully followed to detect local relapse and should also practice self-examination [44].

Radiation Therapy

External beam radiotherapy (EBRT) using megavoltage telecobalt gamma rays or 6 MV photons from linear accelerators or interstitial implantation [28] or surface applicators [45] of radioactive iridium 192 (brachytherapy) has been used successfully in the treatment of early penile cancers for more than 50 years. The type of radiotherapy best suited for a patient depends on the tumor location, size, thickness, and its proximity to the urethra. Small, superficial tumors anywhere over the glans can be treated with surface mold therapy, localized small tumors away from the urethra can be treated with interstitial implant, and any tumor can be adequately treated with EBRT. Although EBRT has universal applicability and can be successfully delivered in all radiotherapy departments, excellent tumor control without severe complications with brachytherapy mandates strict case selection and expertise with the specialized procedure [28]. Thus even for small localized tumors, external radiation may be preferable if the requisite expertise and facilities for penile brachytherapy is not available.

In EBRT, the glans and the distal 2 to 5 cm of penile shaft is irradiated using bilateral megavoltage beams. For immobilization and repositioning of the penis during treatment and for providing surface buildup of radiation dose, a special device such as a wooden jig [30], wax block [45], or transparent Perspex device [31] is used. A transparent device allows visualization of the penis and maximum sparing of the penile shaft in tumors confined to the glans. A variety of fractionation schedules have been described in the literature with variable results. In addition to the conventional fractionation of 60 Gy in 30 daily fractions over 6 weeks [30,31], other hypofractionated accelerated regimens such as 50 to 55 Gy in 16 daily fractions over 3 weeks [46] and 50 to 55 Gy in 20 to 22 daily fractions over 4 weeks [45] have been used. At the Tata Memorial Hospital we traditionally used a hypofractionated accelerated regimen of 55 Gy in 16 daily fractions over 3 weeks. This provided excellent local control in early cancers without any symptomatic late sequelae. However, the acute radiation mucocutaneous reaction over the glans and penile shaft healed after a median period of 12 weeks. After we slightly modified the fractionation to 54 Gy in 18 daily fractions in $3\frac{1}{2}$ weeks, the median healing time for acute reaction has been reduced to 6 weeks, without affecting the tumor control rate. This is comparable to the healing time following laser photocoagulation [37]. The main advantage of the accelerated 3- to 4-week regimen over the more protracted 6-week regimen is that it allows the completion of radiotherapy before the onset of the inevitable brisk radiation reaction. Brisk radiation reaction during radiotherapy can cause treatment interruption of a protracted regimen, and this has been shown to adversely affect tumor control due to tumor repopulation [31].

Local tumor control following radiotherapy is largely determined by the tumor stage, with better results for T1 and selected T2 tumors and universally poor local control in more advanced tumors [28,30–32,47]. Results of brachytherapy series [28,32] are superior to external radiotherapy series [30,31], but this may be largely due to the selective use of brachytherapy for smaller and noninfiltrative tumors. Due to successful surgical salvage, the eventual local control rates are comparable between the implant and EBRT series. However, severe complications such as radiation necrosis requiring penectomy or symptomatic urethral strictures are also higher with brachytherapy (Table 11.3). In the ongoing prospective study of accelerated external radiation at our institute, at a median follow-up of 30 months local recurrence has occurred in only one of 17 patients with tumor confined to the glans as compared to four of six patients with signs of shaft infiltration. All five penile recurrences have been successfully salvaged by partial penectomy. Local failure rates as high as 35% to 40% have been reported in the two largest external radiotherapy series using a more protracted 6-week regimen [30,31]. However, in both these studies, the vast majority of penile recurrences were surgically salvaged, thereby achieving local control in 90% to 98% of patients (Table 11.3). These results support the policy of radical radiotherapy, with surgery reserved for salvage in early-stage disease. The European Board of Urology has endorsed this treatment strategy of organ conserving therapy and watchful waiting for early-stage disease [48]. Because the results of radiotherapy alone are poor in more advanced tumors [30,31], initial penectomy is the treatment of choice for such tumors.

Penile Amputation

Amputation of the penis is the most widely used and undoubtedly the safest treatment approach in all stages of the disease.

Though it has been considered as the gold standard of local treatment by some [3], due to the associated psychosexual dysfunction amputative surgery should be reserved for patients not suitable for PCT due to tumor infiltration or if sexual dysfunction is unlikely do be of concern to the patient, or due to expected noncompliance with close follow-up after PCT.

Partial penectomy is indicated for lesions involving the glans, corona, and distal shaft, where after adequate surgical excision the residual penile stump ensures upright micturition without scrotal soiling and for sexual function. Traditionally, a 2-cm disease-free margin has been advocated. However, Hoffman et al. [49] reported no recurrence in any of their patients with microscopic margins up to 10 mm. Similar findings have also been reported by Agrawal et al. [50], who feel that a 10-mm margin may be adequate for grade I and II lesions and 15 mm for grade III lesions. This approach would qualify more patients for conservative surgery or partial penectomy rather than total penectomy, and the residual penile length would then be cosmetically and functionally more acceptable. Patients undergoing partial penectomy can be offered penile augmentation or reconstructive surgery at a later date, if they wish to have the normal length of the penis restored.

Total penectomy with perineal urethrostomy is indicated when the lesion extends to involve the proximal shaft or the base of the penis. Sometimes, limited extension to the scrotum or the skin overlying the pubis may also require wide excision of these structures. With local spread and bone invasion, local bone resection may also be required. The risk of local recurrence after an appropriate amputative surgery should be negligible [3,6,31,35,37]. Urethra-sparing total or subtotal penectomy followed by delayed penile reconstruction has been reported for invasive penile lesions involving only the dorsum of the penis [51].

Management of Ilioinguinal Nodes

Lymph node metastasis in patients with penile cancer is the main determinant of survival, and optimal management of regional nodes is challenging as well as controversial. Superficial and deep inguinal nodes are the first-echelon nodes, with skip metastasis in the pelvic lymph nodes being very rare. The diagnostic and therapeutic approach for the ilioinguinal nodes depends on the index of suspicion for nodal metastasis in a clinically negative groin, and the laterality, size, and mobility of any clinically manifest nodes.

Impalpable or Clinically Insignificant Groin Nodes

In patients with impalpable or clinically insignificant groin nodes with a negative FNAC, there is no consensus regarding selection of patients for close surveillance, sentinel node biopsy, or groin node dissection. Because clinical examination, imaging, and FNAC may miss subclinical nodal metastasis in up to 20% patients [3,24], special diagnostic procedures such as sentinel node biopsy or limited surgery to identify occult metastases and prophylactic node dissection have been evaluated by various investigators.

Surveillance

Due to the morbidity of prophylactic node dissection, a procedure that will be an overtreatment in 80% of patients, and pitfalls in special diagnostic procedures such as sentinel node biopsy, a policy of close surveillance with node dissection reserved for clinically manifest nodal metastases seems attractive. However, the safety of such a policy is questionable in patients who are at a high risk of harboring subclinical nodal metastases or those who may not comply with a very strict surveillance program. Various clinical and histological parameters can help to stratify patients at an increased risk of harboring occult inguinal nodal metastasis. Tumor size, histological grade, infiltration of the corpora cavernosa and spongiosum, and lymphovascular emboli have been found as the main predictors of occult nodal metastases in most studies [11,13,16–18]. Of these the most important factors are the T status and histological grade, as shown in Table 11.1 and discussed earlier. Thus patients who are at low risk of occult nodal metastases and reliable for close follow-up are ideal candidates for the policy of surveillance and therapeutic lymphadenectomy for metastatic lymphadenopathy detected at follow-up. Delayed therapeutic lymphadenectomy for clinically positive nodes detected during active surveillance does not seem to jeopardize long-term survival [17]. Because most inguinal node metastases occur within 2 to 3 years following initial therapy, the surveillance must cover this period with repeated examinations at 1- to 3-month intervals. In patients with infiltrating or poorly differentiated tumors, the long-term safety of surveillance is not known.

Sentinel Node Biopsy

This approach, which addresses the concern that delayed node dissection may affect survival, has gained credence due to its potential for significantly reducing the morbidity of ilioinguinal lymphadenectomy. Cabanas [52] described sentinel node biopsy (removal of a node in the superomedial to saphenofemoral junction in the region of the superficial epigastric vein) and advocated formal lymph node dissection if the node was proved metastatic. He hypothesized that in the absence of sen-tinel node metastasis, metastasis in the inguinofemoral or iliac nodes is not possible. Scappini et al. [53] suggested aspiration cytology under lymphangiographic guidance. However, a significant false-negative rate of sentinel node biopsy manifesting as subsequent nodal relapse has been noted in several studies [54–56]. However, studies have shown that occult lymph node metastases in penile cancer can be detected with a sensitivity of over 80% by dynamic sentinel node biopsy, including preoperative lymphoscintigraphy, vital dye, and a gamma ray detection probe [57–59]. The dynamic sentinel node procedure is a promising staging technique to detect early metastatic dissemination of penile cancer based on individual mapping of lymphatic drainage, and enables identification of patients with clinically node negative disease requiring regional lymph node dissection [57]. Recently, Lont et al. [60] evaluated the clini-cal outcome of clinically node-nega-tive penile cancers managed by surveillance or further diagnosed by dynamic sentinel node biopsy with subsequent resection of inguinal nodes. They concluded that early detection of lymph node metastases by dynamic sentinel node biopsy and subsequent resection in clinically node negative T2–3 penile cancers improves survival compared with a policy of surveillance (91% vs. 79% at 3 years).

Limited Surgery for Identifying Occult Metastases

Due to significant false-negative rates of sentinel node biopsy noted in a few studies, limited surgery for identifying occult metastases has been evaluated by a number of authors. Senthil

Kumar et al. [61] evaluated the relative value of FNAC, sentinel node biopsy, and medial inguinal node biopsy. They concluded that FNAC is accurate and specific if the nodes are palpable; if the nodes are impalpable, a preliminary medial inguinal node biopsy followed by sentinel node biopsy if medial inguinal node biopsy is negative will accurately select all patients with metastases in the groin nodes. Superficial or modified inguinal lymphadenectomy followed by a deep inguinal and pelvic lymphadenectomy if superficial nodes are positive on frozen section avoids the pitfalls of sentinel node biopsy without significantly increasing the morbidity [19,62].

Prophylactic Lymphadenectomy

Early adjunctive prophylactic lymphadenectomy has been employed in patients who on the basis of the clinical and histological criteria discussed earlier are considered to be at a high risk of harboring occult metastasis. When prophylactic lymphadenectomy is being performed with the aim of curing patients who may have occult metastasis, one has to bear in mind the likely survival benefit and morbidity attributable to the procedure. The cure rates after inguinal lymphadenectomy in the presence of limited nodal metastasis may be as high as 80%. The proponents of lymphadenectomy in patients with clinically nonpalpable inguinal nodes claim that because the curative benefit of lymphadenectomy in the presence of palpable metastatic nodes is well established, it seems logical that lymphadenectomy performed in the setting of occult nodal disease would confer an even greater advantage. Some authors have reported a significant reduction in survival in patients undergoing delayed therapeutic rather than prophylactic lymphadenectomy, thereby suggesting that the best results can be obtained in the presence of a low tumor load [16,63,64] and that delaying lymphadenectomy may be inappropriate [16,17,35,65,66]. Some earlier studies, however, did not find any significant adverse impact on survival of a delayed therapeutic groin node dissection for metastatic nodes on follow-up, with survival rates equivalent to those obtained with initial therapeutic lymphadenectomy for metastatic nodes at presentation [67–69]. These studies, however, reported on lymphadenectomy for clinically palpable nodal disease and do not exclude the possibility that lymphadenectomy for clinically occult nodes may yield a better survival. Randomized trials proving the

23. Vapnek JM, Hricak H, Carroll PR. Recent advances in imaging studies for staging of penile and urethral carcinoma. Urol Clin North Am 1992;19:257–266.

24. Ravi R. Correlation between the extent of nodal involvement and survival following groin dissection for carcinoma of the penis. Br J Urol 1993;72:817–819.

25. Jackson SM. The treatment of carcinoma of the penis. Br J Surg 1966;53:33–35.

26. Horenblas S, Van Tinteren H. Squamous cell carcinoma of the penis. IV. Prognostic factors of survival: analysis of tumor, nodes and metastasis classification system. J Urol 1994;151:1239–1243.

27. Harden SV, Tan LT. Treatment of localized carcinoma of the penis: a survey of current practice in the UK. Clin Oncol (R Coll Radiol) 2001;13:284–287.

28. Rozan R, Albuisson E, Giraud B, et al. Interstitial brachytherapy for penile carcinoma: a multicentric survey (259 patients). Radiother Oncol 1995;36:83–93.

29. Delannes M, Malavaud B, Douchez J, Bonnet J, Daly NJ. Iridium-192 interstitial therapy for squamous cell carcinoma of the penis. Int J Radiat Oncol Biol Phys 1992;24:479–483.

30. Ravi R, Chaturvedi HK, Sastry DVLN. Role of radiation therapy in the treatment of carcinoma of the penis. Br J Urol 1994;74:646–651.

31. Sarin R, Norman AR, Steel GG, Horwich A. Treatment results and prognostic factors in 101 men treated for squamous carcinoma of the penis. Int J Radiat Oncol Biol Phys 1997;38:713–722.

32. Chaudhary AJ, Ghosh S, Bhalavat RL, Kulkarni JN, Sequeira BV. Interstitial brachytherapy in carcinoma of the penis. Strahlenther Onkol 1999;175:17–20.

33. Narayana AS, Olney LE, Loening SA, Weimar G, Culp DA. Carcinoma of the penis: analysis of 219 cases. Cancer 1982;49:2185–2191.

34. Hardner GJ, Bhanalaph T, Murphy GP, Albert DJ, Moore RH. Carcinoma of the penis: analysis of therapy in 100 consecutive cases. J Urol 1972;108:428–430.

35. McDougal WS, Kirchner FK Jr, Edwards RH, Killon LT. Treatment of carcinoma of the penis: the case of primary lymphadenectomy. J Urol 1986;136:38–41.

36. Jensen MS. Cancer of the penis in Denmark 1942 to 1962 (511 cases). Dan Med Bull 1977;24:66–72.

37. Horenblas S, Van Tinteren H, Delemare JFM. Squamous cell carcinoma of the penis: treatment of the primary tumour. J Urol 1992;147:1533–1538.

38. Mohs FE, Snow SN, Messing EM, Kuglitsch ME. Microscopically controlled surgery in the treatment of carcinoma of the penis. J Urol 1985;133:961–966.

39. Brown MD, Zachary CB, Grekin RC, Swanson NA. Penile tumors: their management by Mohs micrographic surgery. J Dermatol Surg Oncol 1987;13:1163–1167.

40. Bandiermonte, Santoro O, Boracchi P, Piva L, Pizzocaro G, DePalo G. Total resection of glans penis surface by CO2 laser microsurgery. Acta Oncol 1988;27:575–578.

41. Rothenberger KH. Value of the neodymium YAG laser in the therapy of penile carcinoma. Eur Urol 1986;12(suppl 1):34–36.

42. Windahl T, Andersson SO. Combined laser treatment for penile carcinoma: results after long-term followup. J Urol 2003;169:2118–2121.

43. Frimberger D, Hungerhuber E, Zaak D, Waidelich R, Hofstetter A, Schneede P. Penile carcinoma. Is Nd:YAG laser therapy radical enough? J Urol 2002;168:2418–2421.

44. Van Bezooijen BP, Horenblas S, Meinhardt W, Newling DW. Laser therapy for carcinoma in situ of the penis. J Urol 2001;166: 670–671.

45. Neave F, Neal AJ, Hoskin PJ, Hope-Stone HF. Carcinoma of the penis: a retrospective review of treatment with iridium mould and external beam irradiation. Clin Oncol 1993;5:207–210.

46. Duncan W, Jackson SM. Treatment of early cancer of penis with megavoltage x-rays. Clin Radiol 1972;23:246–248.

47. Modig H, Duchek M, Sjodin JG. Carcinoma of the penis. Treatment by surgery or combined bleomycin and radiation therapy. Acta Oncol 1993;32:653–655.

48. Lindegaard JC, Nielsen OS, Lundbeck FA, Mamsen A, Studstrup HN, von der Maase H. A retrospective analysis of 82 cases of cancer of the penis. Br J Urol 1996;77:883–890.

49. Hoffman MA, Renshaw AA, Loughlin KR. Squamous cell carcinoma of the penis and microscopic pathologic margins: how much margin is needed for local cure? Cancer. 1999;85:1565–1568.

50. Agrawal A, Pai D, Ananthakrishnan N, Smile SR, Ratnakar C. The histological extent of the local spread of carcinoma of the penis and its therapeutic implications. BJU Int 2000;85:299–301.

51. Bissada NK, Morcos RR, El-Senoussi M. Post-circumcision carcinoma of the penis. I. Clinical aspects. J Urol 1986;135:283–285.

52. Cabanas RM. An approach for the treatment of penile carcinoma. Cancer 1977;39:456–466.

53. Scappini P, Piscioli F, Pusiol T, Hofstetter A, Rothenberger KH, Luciani L. Penile cancer: aspiration biopsy cytology for staging. Cancer 1986;58:1526–1533.

54. Perinetti EP, Crane DC, Catalona WJ. Unreliability of sentinel node biopsy for staging penile carcinoma. J Urol 1980;124:734–735.

55. Pettaway CA, Pisters LL, Dinney CP, et al. Sentinel lymph node dissection for penile carcinoma: the M. D. Anderson Cancer Center experience. J Urol 1995;154:1999–2003.

56. Valdes Olmos RA, Tanis PJ, Hoefnagel CA, et al. Penile lymphoscintigraphy for sentinel node identification. Eur J Nucl Med 2001;28:581–585.

57. Horenblas S, Jansen L, Meinhardt W, Hoefnagel CA, de Jong D, Nieweg OE. Detection of occult metastasis in squamous cell carcinoma of the penis using a dynamic sentinel node procedure. J Urol 2000;163:100–104.

58. Han KR, Brogle BN, Goydos J, Perrotti M, Cummings KB, Weiss RE. Lymphatic mapping and intraoperative lymphoscintigraphy for identifying the sentinel node in penile tumors. Urology 2000;55: 582–585.

59. Tanis PJ, Lont AP, Meinhardt W, Olmos RA, Nieweg OE, Horenblas S. Dynamic sentinel node biopsy for penile cancer: reliability of a staging technique. J Urol 2002;168:76–80.

60. Lont AP, Horenblas S, Tanis PJ, Gallee MP, van Tinteren H, Nieweg OE. Management of clinically node negative penile carcinoma: improved survival after the introduction of dynamic sentinel node biopsy. J Urol 2003;170:783–786.

61. Senthil Kumar MP, Ananthakrishnan N, Prema V. Predicting regional lymph node metastasis in carcinoma of penis: a comparison between fine needle aspiration cytology, sentinel lymph node biopsy and medial inguinal lymph node biopsy. Br J Urol 1998;81:453–457.

62. Sanchez-Oritz RF, Pettaway CA. Natural history, management, and surveillance of recurrent squamous cell penile carcinoma: a risk based approach. Urol Clin North Am 2003;30:853–867.

63. Srinivas V, Morse MJ, Herr HW, Sogani PC, Whitmore WF Jr. Penile cancer: relation of extent of nodal metastasis to survival. J Urol 1987;137:880–882.

64. Fossa SD, Hall KS, Johannessen NB, Urnes T, Kaalhus O. Cancer of the penis. Experience at the Norwegian Radium Hospital 1974–1985. Eur Urol 1987;13:372–377.

65. Ornellas AA, Seixas LC, Marota A. Surgical treatment of invasive squamous cell carcinoma of the penis: retrospective analysis of 350 cases. J Urol 1994;151:1244–1249.

66. Johnson DE, Lo RK. Management of regional lymph nodes in penile carcinoma: five year results following therapeutic groin dissections. Urology 1984;24:308–311.

67. Beggs JH, Spratt JS. Epidermoid carcinoma of the penis. J Urol 1961;91:166–172.

68. Frew ID, Jefferies JD, Swinney J. Carcinoma of penis. Br J Urol 1967;39:398–404.

69. Baker BH, Spratt JS, Perez-Mesa C. Carcinoma of the penis. J Urol 1976;116:458–461.

70. Tongaonkar HB, Kulkarni JN, Kamat MR. Carcinoma of the penis: relationship of nodal metastases to survival. Indian J Urol 1993;9:54–57.

71. Gursel EO, Georgountzos C, Uson AC, Melicow MM, Veenema RJ. Penile cancer. Urology 1973;1:569–578.
72. Assimos DG, Jarow JP. Role of laparoscopic pelvic lymph node dissection in the management of patients with penile cancer and inguinal adenopathy. J Endourol 1994;8:365–369.
73. Fraley EE, Hutchens HC. Radical ilio-inguinal node dissection: the skin bridge technique. A new procedure. J Urol 1972;108:279–281.
74. Catalona WJ. Modified inguinal lymphadenectomy for carcinoma of the penis with preservation of saphenous veins: technique and preliminary results. J Urol 1988;140:306–310.
75. Coblentz TR, Theodorescu D. Morbidity of modified prophylactic inguinal lymphadenectomy for squamous cell carcinoma of the penis. J Urol 2002;168:1386–1389.
76. Jacobellis U. Modified radical inguinal lymphadenectomy for carcinoma of the penis: technique and results. J Urol 2003;169:1349–1352.
77. Savant DN, Dalal AV, Patel SG, Bhathena HM, Kavarana NM. Tensor fasciae lata myocutaneous flap reconstruction following ilioinguinal node dissection. Eur J Plast Surg 1996;19:174–177.
78. Goette DK, Carson TE. Erythroplasia of Queyrat: treatment with topical 5–fluorouracil. Cancer 1976;38:1498–1502.
79. Schroeder TL, Sengelmann RD. Squamous cell carcinoma in situ of the penis successfully treated with imiquimod 5% cream. J Am Acad Dermatol 2002;46:545–548.
80. Culkin DJ, Beer TM. Advanced penile carcinoma. J Urol 2003;170:359–365.
81. Hussein AM, Benedetto P, Sridhar KS. Chemotherapy with cisplatin and 5-fluorouracil for penile and urethral squamous cell carcinomas. Cancer 1990;65:433–438.
82. Shammas FV, Ous S, Fossa SD. Cisplatin and 5-fluorouracil in advanced cancer of the penis. J Urol 1992;147:630–632.
83. Haas GP, Blumenstein BA, Gagliano RG, et al. Cisplatin, methotrexate and bleomycin for the treatment of carcinoma of the penis: a Southwest Oncology Group study. J Urol 1999;161:1823–1825.
84. Pizzocaro G, Piva L, Bandieramonte G, Tana S. Up-to-date management of carcinoma of the penis. Eur Urol 1997;32:5–15.
85. Kattan J, Culine S, Droz JP, et al. Penile cancer chemotherapy: twelve years' experience at Institut Gustave-Roussy. Urology 1993;42:559–562.
86. Rozan R, Albuisson E, Giraud B, Boiteux JP, Dauplat J. Epithelioma of the penis treated with surgery. Study Group on Urogenital Tumors of the National Federation of the Centers for Cancer Control. Prog Urol 1996;6:926–935.
87. Lindegaard JC, Nielsen OS, Lundbeck FA, Mamsen A, Studstrup HN, von der Maase H. A retrospective analysis of 82 cases of cancer of the penis. Br J Urol 1996;77:883–890.

88. Opjordsmoen S, Waehre H, Aass N, Fossa SD. Sexuality in patients treated for penile cancer: patient's experience and doctor's judgement. Br J Urol 1994;73:554–560.
89. Ficarra V, Mofferdin A, D'Amico A, et al. Comparison of the quality of life of patients treated by surgery or radiotherapy in epidermoid cancer of the penis. Prog Urol 1999;9:715–720.
90. Munro NP, Thomas PJ, Deutsch GP, Hodson NJ. Penile cancer: a case for guidelines. Ann R Coll Surg Engl 2001;83:180–185.

Index

benefit of prophylactic over delayed therapeutic lymphadenec-tomy are needed to incorporate routine prophylactic lym-phadenectomy into clinical practice. Moreover, the significant early and delayed morbidity of the lymphadenectomy and the lack of therapeutic benefit in nearly 75% of patients undergoing this procedure has prevented routine prophylactic lymphade-nectomy from being the standard treatment for all patients with clinically nonpalpable nodes.

Clinically Significant or Cytologically Confirmed Groin Nodes

In patients with operable nodes, surgery is the mainstay of treat-ment and often curative, especially for those with limited nodal metastasis. In planning the most appropriate treatment, these patients should be evaluated clinically for operability and with a contrast-enhanced CT scan, especially for pelvic nodes. Various authors have reported that 20% to 67% of patients with clinically palpable metastatic inguinal lymph node metastasis will be disease free at 5 years after lymphadenectomy [35,63–67]. The extent and level of lymph node metastases have been shown to be important predictors of survival [16,24,63–67,70].

Extent of Lymphadenectomy

Bilateral ilioinguinal lymphadenectomy is mandatory for patients with bilateral lymph node metastases. Bilateral lymphadenec-tomy is also recommended for patients with unilateral significant lymphadenopathy at presentation because clinically occult con-tralateral groin metastases can be present in over 50% of such patients [54,75]. Node dissection on the contralateral side may be limited to superficial node dissection if no histological evidence of metastasis is found in the contralateral superficial nodes. In patients who develop metachronous unilateral lymph node metastasis while on surveillance, it may be sufficient to perform a unilateral lymph node dissection, especially if the metastasis-free interval is longer than 1 year. This is especially so because the patients selected for surveillance have a very low rate (appro-ximately 10%) of metachronous metastasis, and the chance of developing contralateral node metastasis subsequently is extremely low. Enlarged metastatic groin nodes that are adherent to the overlying skin or ulcerating through it require wide excision of the skin around the node mass, with closure of the consequent skin defect using myocutaneous flap.

Modified or extended sentinel node dissection also has been advocated for patients with limited inguinal node disease in order to reduce the morbidity of radical ilioinguinal lymphadenectomy. However, one study reported that five of the 14 patients who underwent a therapeutic modified superficial inguinal dissection relapsed with incurable groin metastases within 2 years [55]. Hence, radical ilioinguinal lymphadenectomy is the procedure of choice in patients with metastatic nodes.

The therapeutic benefit of pelvic lymphadenectomy in the presence of metastatic inguinal nodes is still undetermined. Iliac lymph node metastases are found in approximately 15% to 30% of patients with metastatic inguinal lymph nodes [63,71], the incidence being higher for a greater number of positive inguinal lymph nodes, presence of perinodal extension, and bilaterality of disease [24,63]. Although Srinivas et al. [63] reported that none of their 11 patients with iliac lymph node metastasis survived 3 years, others have reported fair survival with positive pelvic nodes [52], with improvement in survival documented after iliac node dissection [34]. Lopes et al. [19], in their small series, reported that ilioinguinal lymphadenectomy may have a significant role in increasing the survival of patients with metastases to only one iliac lymph node. In view of this, it seems reasonable to extend the lymph node dissection to include the iliac nodes. A laparoscopic approach may also be used to complete the pelvic node dissection [72].

Complications of Ilioinguinal Lymphadenectomy

Although perioperative mortality consequent to ilioinguinal lymphadenectomy is rare, the morbidity of the procedure is quite significant. Skin flap or edge necrosis and wound breakdown along with persistent lymphorrhea are the commonest early complications reported in up to 80% of patients [65,66]. This may lead to prolonged hospitalization or may require secondary reconstruction with skin grafts or pedicled flaps. Routine transposition of the sartorius muscle to cover the femoral vessels has almost completely eliminated the risk of femoral vessel blowout. The commonest delayed complication is debilitating lower extremity or penoscrotal lymphedema seen in nearly one third of patients. In light of this, a lot of attention has recently focused on reduction of morbidity by modification of the surgical procedure.

Modifications of surgical incisions have been explored at a number of centres. Fraley and Hutchens [73] employed two parallel incisions in the groin, one above and one below the inguinal ligament to reduce the skin flap or edge necrosis. Similarly, a technique of a transverse incision below the inguinal ligament for the inguinal lymphadenectomy and a midline infraumbilical incision for bilateral extraperitoneal pelvic node dissection has been described with significant reduction in the skin loss. However, the choice of incision has little or no bearing on the lower extremity edema. The technique of saphen-ous vein preserving modified inguinal lymphadenectomy was first described by Catalona [74], with consequent reduction in the incidence of debilitating limb edema. He also redefined the lateral boundary of the dissection as the femoral artery and dispensed with the mobilization and transposition of the sartorius muscle. Iliac node dissection was also not carried out in the absence of inguinal nodal metastases. These modifications seemed suitable in patients with negative inguinal nodes and resulted in reduction in the rate of wound breakdown and skin loss to less than 20%. This saphenous vein–sparing approach has gained credibility especially in patients undergoing prophylactic lymphadenectomy. Coblentz and Theodorescu [75] also employed the saphenous vein–sparing approach along with thick skin flaps during prophylactic inguinal lymphadenectomy for high-risk disease. Early follow-up of their patients indicates that the nodal control rates are comparable to those in similar patients reported in the literature treated with classic lymphadenectomy technique. However, the value of these modifications in the context of metastatic lymphadenopathy, which warrants a complete radical lymphadenectomy, is questionable.

Jacobellis [76] described a technique of modified radical inguinal lymphadenectomy, wherein to avoid damage to the vessels of the groin region that run parallel to the inguinal ligament and lie in the fat of the superficial layer of the superficial fascia, dissection is done beneath this layer (deep to Scarpa's fascia), he saphenous nerve is preserved and the sartorius is left in situ so as not to disturb the collateral lymphatic drainage. He reported no skin necrosis, infection, or deep vein thrombosis, and only moderate lymphedema in four patients at a follow up of 6 to 104 months in his series of 10 patients.

At the Tata Memorial Hospital, we practice routine excision of the skin overlying the inguinal nodal area in all patients undergoing radical ilioinguinal lymphadenectomy, even when the skin is not infiltrated by the nodal disease and we perform immediate reconstruction using a tensor fascia lata myocutaneous flap or anterolateral thigh flap [70,77]. We have had no major problems of skin loss or wound breakdown since the time we began employing this procedure. In addition, the incidence of lower extremity lymphedema has also been significantly reduced with a long follow-up in these patients. With the majority of patients having no significant physical impairment and with preservation of a good quality of life, this may represent a significant advance in the reduction of morbidity of ilioinguinal lymphadenectomy. Alternatives to these flaps are the rectus abdominis flap or the gracilis flap.

Chemotherapy

Chemotherapy for penile cancer has been evaluated in two distinct clinical settings. Topical application of 5-fluorouracil cream [78] and more recently imiquimod 5% cream [79] has been found useful in selected patients with carcinoma-in-situ [1]. There are very few studies of systemic chemotherapy in invasive penile cancer. In early invasive T1–2 N0 penile can-cer, concurrent daily bleomycin chemotherapy regimen with radiotherapy has been reported to show a local control rate of 80%. However, with good results of modern radiotherapy alone, there is no role for chemotherapy along with radiotherapy in early-stage disease now. Review of the published literature reveals that cisplatin-based chemotherapy is the most commonly used regimen in advanced penile cancer [80], with nearly 70% response rates. It seems to allow approximately 40% patients with regionally disseminated penile cancer to undergo complete inguinal lymphadenectomy and about 23% to achieve a durable long-term disease-free survival [81–85]. In a Southwest Oncology Group study, 45 patients with locally advanced or metastatic penile carcinoma, were treated with cisplatin $75 \, mg/m^2$ day 1, methotrexate $25 \, mg/m^2$ days 1 and 8, and bleomycin $10 \, U/m^2$ on days 1 and 8 with a cycle length of 21 days. Although the response rate was only 32%, five toxic deaths and six life-threatening toxic episodes were seen [83].

Prognosis

In patients with early-stage disease, there are few deaths due to penile cancer and the long-term overall survival rates are often determined by the comorbid conditions in an elderly population [28,31,86]. Depending on the proportion of cases in different stages, 5-year penile cancer–specific survival rates of 66% to 88% have been reported [28,31,86]. Of the few large studies with multivariate analysis of prognostic factors, nodal metastases [9,19,31], higher T stage or invasion [9,31,48], and high histological grade [31,48] were identified as independent adverse prognostic factors for survival. The substratification of nodal status such as three or more nodes, bilateral disease, extranodal extension, and iliac node metastases predict an especially poor prognosis [6,24,34,63,65].

Quality of Life and Psychosexual Issues

These issues, unfortunately, have been entirely neglected in most reports on penile cancer. This is surprising considering the possible major psychosexual impact of a penectomy. There are only a few small, mostly retrospective studies evaluating the quality of life and psychosexual issues (2,88,89). The expected quality of life, particularly sexual functions after treatment, should be specifically discussed with the patient. It is an expansive concept that involves vast and profound evaluation. The Overall Sexual Functioning Questionnaire (OSFQ), first used by Opjordsmoen et al. [2,87], is a useful tool and should be used to assess sexual quality of life before and after treatment (Table 11.4). This tool can be very useful to compare different treatment modalities like surgery and radiotherapy in deciding the best approach for early cancers. In a Norwegian study [88] moderate to severe sexual dysfunction was observed in only two of 10 patients after radiotherapy compared to four of five after wide excision, seven of nine after partial penectomy, and all four after total penectomy. We have previously reported that of the 29 patients treated with penectomy, one committed suicide and another had a failed

Table 11.4. Overall Sexual Functioning Questionnaire (OSFQ) [2,87]

Parameter	Score
1. Sexual interest	0 (No sexual interest) to 4 (normal)
2. Sexual ability	0 (Lack of ability) to 4 (no problems)
3. Sexual satisfaction	1 (lacking) to 4 (no change)
4. Relationship with partner	1 (very distressed) to 4 (unchanged, good)
5. Sexual identity	2 (very much changed) to 4 (normal)
6. Frequency of coitus	1 (no sexual intercourse) to 4 (no reduction)

Global score of overall sexual function (five categories).
  I No sexual functioning score, 5–8.
 II Severely reduced score, 9–14.
III Moderately reduced score, 15–19.
IV Slightly reduced score, 20–22.
 V Normal score, 23–24.

suicide attempt [31]. In an Italian study of 17 patients treated with amputative surgery, anxiety was evident in 30% and depression was evident in one patient, and the global sexual function was compromised in 76% [89].

In our ongoing prospective study of accelerated radiotherapy at the Tata Memorial Hospital, of the 18 patients with intact penis (five underwent penectomy for residual/recurrent disease), 16 men have retained their pretreatment erectile function, coital satisfaction, and frequency. The remaining two patients have reported mild sexual dysfunction after radiotherapy.

Conclusion

Penile cancers, though uncommon in developed countries, pose a significant oncological challenge in some parts of the world. With the available treatment options, the aim of treatment should be organ and function preservation whenever possible, without compromising the chances of survival. Early-stage cancers in men who wish to preserve organ and function and are expected to be compliant with a close follow-up program should be offered an appropriate penile conservative therapy. More advanced tumors are difficult to control with radiotherapy; hence

Printed in Singapore